"*Even having grown up in town and as an avid runner, walker, and cyclist, I learned of so many secret passageways. I also loved the history.*"

—Claire Gallogly, Transportation planner

"*I was thrilled to read this book of walks to find that I at once felt more deeply connected to the Santa Cruz I know so well and also excited to learn about the hidden gems of history, nature and secret paths that feel like new adventures awaiting me.*"

—Theresia Rogerson, Public health professional

"*A must read for those new to Santa Cruz. A great guide for those who have lived here for years.*"

— Katherine Beiers, Former Mayor of Santa Cruz

"*As a car-free resident of Santa Cruz for 45 years, I nevertheless encountered a couple of surprise walkways and was reacquainted with several other forgotten gems as I followed the delightful routes in this book. And being very well written, format-ted and illustrated, it will entice even first-timers to our area to discover and enjoy the many diverse and inspiring jaunts presented.*"

— Rick Hyman, Environmental planner, bicycle advocate

"*Read this book, and try walking on their routes. You will get good exercise, and you will learn about where you are.*"

—Peter Scott, Transportation activist

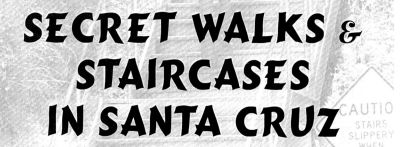

SECRET WALKS & STAIRCASES IN SANTA CRUZ

CAUTION
STAIRS
SLIPPERY
WHEN
WET

28
WALKS
FOR FUN
AND
FITNESS

DEBBIE BULGER & RICHARD STOVER

first edition
sixth printing
https://www.lostballoonpress.com
Printed in Santa Cruz, CA, United States of America

Book design and layout: Debbie Bulger
Cover design: Debbie Bulger
Photographs: Richard Stover and Debbie Bulger
Maps: Richard Stover

Library of Congress Control Number: 2020919572
ISBN Number 978-0-9899250-1-3

Lost Balloon Press

orders@lostballoonpress.com

Scan this code to reach Lost Balloon Press website.

For Jen and Suzie

A note about the photographs

Photos on the pages before each chapter are of plants and animals one might see on the following walk. Santa Cruz is blessed with having a diversity of natural habitats which support a large number of plant and animal species—some found nowhere else in the world. Below is an example: The Globe Lily, a delicate flower often seen in spring along the Spring Trail in Pogonip.

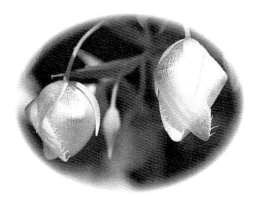

Globe Lily

CONTENTS

Continued on next page

ACKNOWLEDGEMENTS

This book was made clearer and more user friendly by the efforts of several on-the-ground "testers" who each took multiple walks and offered corrections, edits, and suggestions. Comments such as "I think you meant left instead of right," and "be sure to mention the poison oak" are some examples of their input. Especially valuable were the suggestions about omissions in the descriptions. Thank you Medwin Schreher, Carmelita Austin-Schreher, Deborah Benham, G. Severin Marthe, Rick Hyman and family members Jennifer Jackson, Michael Jackson, Suzie Bulger Silverman, Kasey Hegelein, Veronica Hegelein, Barbara Lenox, Sierra Silverman, and Toby Jackson for testing the walks.

We want to give a shout out to local historians Sandy Lydon and Geoff Dunn for their classes which we have taken over the years which helped fill our need to learn about local history after we moved to Santa Cruz in the 1980s. And many thanks to Ross Gibson for answering questions and sharing historic resources.

Suzie Bulger Silverman checked the accuracy of the bird references and helped with proofreading as did Miriam Selig.

Useful feedback on the almost completed manuscript was provided by Katherine Beiers, Theresia Rogerson, Claire Gallogly and Peter Scott.

Special thanks goes to Rick Hyman who not only tested walks on the ground, but also did a final edit of the manuscript. His planning background coupled with his knowledge of local history and hidden byways all resulted in helpful suggestions that made this a more useful book.

Thank you all.

REPORT PEDESTRIAN HAZARDS

Having problems walking because bushes are overgrown or debris is on the sidewalk? You can help solve the problem.

TO REPORT A PROBLEM FOR WALKERS

- Fill out the electronic form at
  sccrtc.org/services/hazard-reports

- Typical problems include overgrown bushes and lack of sidewalks.

- The Santa Cruz County Regional Transportation Commission forwards your report to the appropriate jurisdiction for remedy.

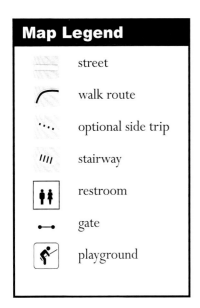

Map Legend

	street
	walk route
	optional side trip
	stairway
	restroom
	gate
	playground

PREFACE

Welcome to *Secret Walks & Staircases in Santa Cruz*. This book is the product of more than 30 years of walking around the community having lived in multiple locations over the years. What began as an evening walk after work turned into walking for errands and finally walking as our main means of transportation.

In the process we came across unmarked staircases, hidden trails at the end of cul-de-sacs and interesting pedestrian shortcuts.

This book is a means of sharing the pleasures of walking with others. As we walk, we note places of historic interest and local birds. Bird sightings are just one of the dividends of travelling quietly by foot. Sauntering rather than speeding in a vehicle enables one to see and examine interesting plants along the way. Walking opens up these interests and many more to the pedestrian. Footnotes are included to assist those who want to delve more deeply into a particular subject.

The book is organized by areas of the community including Eastside, Westside, Downtown, near the Wharf, and more. Each walk is rated by distance and elevation gain to help you decide which ones are right for you and your family. For longer walks we often have an early return option. For the most energetic we have included suggestions of linking walks for a longer experience.

The walks traverse several large parks in Santa Cruz. It is hoped that the short stretches on park trails included here will encourage readers to explore these parks more. Trail guides to the many parks in the area are available online and from various parks departments.

In all this book took six years to complete. Planning took about a year. We created a list of features such as hidden passageways we wanted to share and built walks around the features. We checked each walk on the ground and adjusted routes. As the number of walks grew, the project became more complicated, and it became difficult to keep track of individual routes. To help visualize the book structure we plotted the walks on a foamboard map using colored yarn and pins. Testing continued as the routes came together. We walked each route multiple times, clipboard and GPS in hand to document features, distance and elevation gain. Then we enlisted the help of friends to test whether the directions were clear and if additional points of interest should be added. It was a thorough process which hopfully you will participate in as you use the book.

What is walking?

Walking is fun, fitness, and exploration. Walking is really seeing the world around you.

Walking is transportation.

It is our hope that readers understand that walking is transportation. If people are to successfully deal with Climate Change, we will have to drastically change our behavior regarding travel.

Walking can greatly reduce one's carbon footprint. Walking can be one's primary mode of transportation for trips under one mile and, for many of us, trips under two miles. As the walks in this book show, it can be enjoyable to walk instead of drive to a nearby destination.

We are looking forward to hearing from you, the reader, as you use this book for your walking adventures. Streets change; new paths and trails are built. When you note such new routes, please contact us at
www.lostballoonpress.com
to point out your observations, corrections, and suggestions for additional walks.

—Debbie Bulger and Richard Stover
  Santa Cruz, California, fall 2020

Opposite: Anthony Stairs, North Pacific Avenue

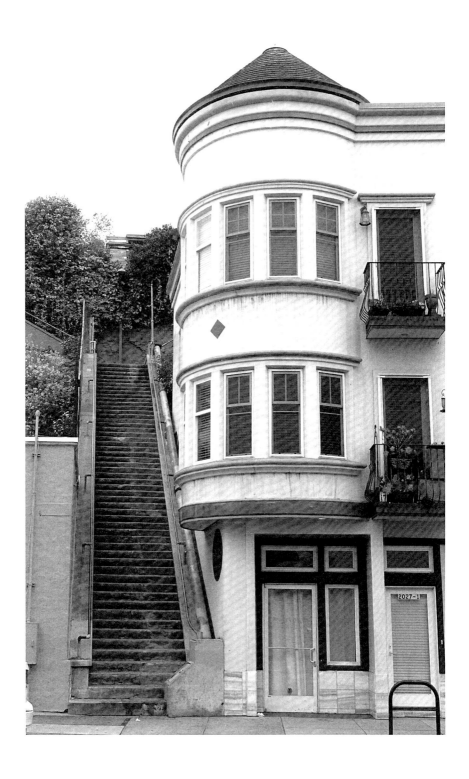

LINKING WALKS

Many of these walks can be linked together for those who want to extend their excursion. Below is a list of pairings much like wine and cheese for your peripatetic pleasure:

DOWNTOWN

Walks 6 & 5:   Downtown + Metro Ctr to Ocean View Ave. = 5.2 miles

Walks 12 & 4:   North Riverwalk + Branciforte Creek Path = 5.7 miles

Walks 1 & 2:   Town Clock + City Hall—Pogonip = 8.6 miles

WESTSIDE

Walks 20 & 21:   Natural Bridge + Long Marine Lab = 5 miles

Walks 20 & 17:   Natural Bridges + Woodrow Ave./Derby Park = 5.9 miles

Walks 10 & 15:   Neary Lagoon + Bay Street—Cowell Ranch = 6.1 miles

WHARF AREA

Walks 7 & 9:   Wharf Itself + Beach Hill = 2.5 miles

Walks 13 & 9:   South Riverwalk + Beach Hill = 3.1 miles

Walks 7 & 8:   Wharf Itself + Wharf to Seabright to Beach Flats = 4 miles

EASTSIDE

Walks 23 & 25:   Arana Gulch—Jose Avenue County Park + East Harbor to Arana Gulch = 5.9 miles

Walks 24 & 23:   Walton Lighthouse + Arana Gulch—Jose Avenue County Park = 6.7 miles

Doubtless you can think of many more combinations. Enjoy the adventure.

WHICH WALK IS RIGHT FOR YOU?
WALKS BY DISTANCE

UNDER TWO MILES

Wharf Itself . . . . 1 mile
Schwan Lake Loops . . . . 1.1 miles
Neary Lagoon Loop . . . . 1.3 miles
Beach Hill . . . . 1.5 miles
Downtown, a Walkable Community . . . . 1.5 miles
South Riverwalk Loop . . . . 1.6 miles

TWO TO FOUR MILES

North Riverwalk Loop . . . . 2.2 miles
East West Cliff to Lighthouse Field semi loop . . . . 2.2 miles
Natural Bridges . . . . 2.3 miles
Town Clock—Anthony Stairs Loop . . . . 2.3 miles
East Cliff Moran Lake Loop . . . . 2.4 miles
East Harbor to Arana Gulch . . . . 2.6 miles
Lighthouse Point to Circles Loop . . . . 2.6 miles
Long Marine Lab—Antonelli Pond . . . . 2.7 miles
Wharf to Seabright to Beach Flats Garden . . . . 3 miles
Wilder Ranch . . . . 3.2 miles
Arana Gulch—Jose Avenue County Park . . . . 3.3 miles
Walton Lighthouse/ Natural History Museum . . . . 3.4 miles
Abbott Square—Harvey West Loop . . . . 3.5 miles
Branciforte Creek Path . . . . 3.5 miles
Woodrow Avenue to Derby Park Loop . . . . 3.6 miles
Metro Center to Ocean View Avenue . . . . 3.7 miles
Both Riverwalk Loops . . . . 3.8 miles
Arroyo Seco—Arboretum . . . . 3.9 miles

OVER FOUR MILES

Bay Street—Cowell Ranch Loop . . . . 4.8 miles
West Cliff to the end and back . . . . 5 miles
Branciforte—DeLaveaga . . . . 5.4 miles
City Hall—Pogonip Loop . . . . 6.3 miles

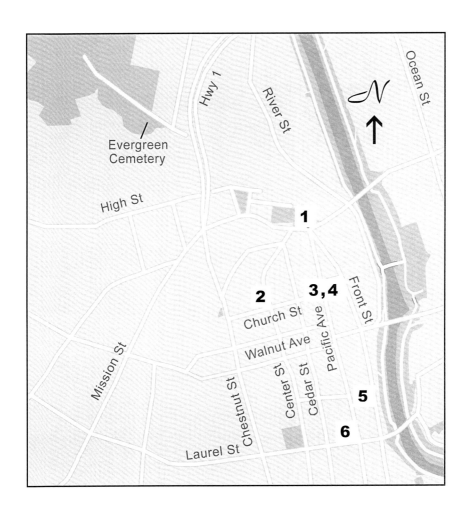

Evergreen
Cemetery

Ocean St

Hwy 1

River St

N

High St

1

2   3,4   Front St

Church St

Pacific Ave

Walnut Ave

Mission St

Chestnut St

Center St

Cedar St

5

6

Laurel St

STARTING FROM DOWNTOWN

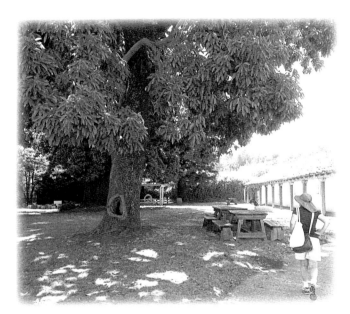

Mission grounds with 100-year-old Avocado Tree.

1 TOWN CLOCK—ANTHONY STAIRS LOOP

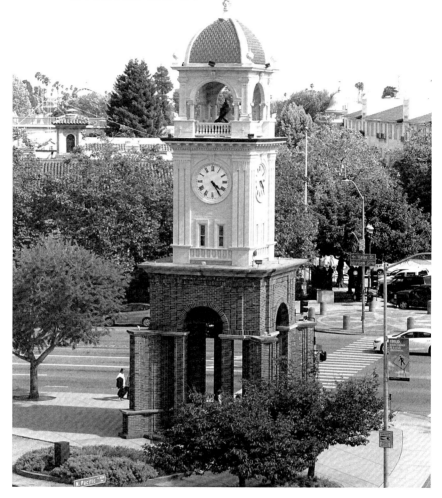

2.3 miles / 170 feet elevation gain

WALK SUMMARY:

The Town Clock is an important gathering place for local demonstrations and silent vigils. Its prominent position at the corner of Pacific/Front/Water Streets makes it an ideal spot

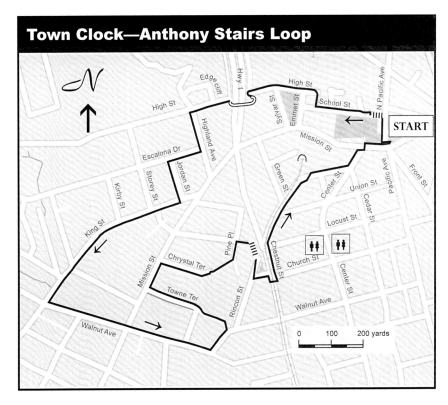

Town Clock—Anthony Stairs Loop

to wave signs at passing drivers and pedestrians. The 1900 Seth Thomas clock originally stood on the top of the IOOF Building (Independent Order of Odd Fellows) nearby on Pacific Avenue and was removed in 1964 when the building was renovated. A new base was erected for the clock in its present location, and the edifice dedicated in 1976. During the Loma Prieta earthquake in 1989, the clock hands stopped at 5:04 p.m.

The sculpture Collateral Damage by local artist E. A. Chase in the small plaza below the clock is a compelling depiction of the horrors of war. The concrete base of the statue contains guns turned in by residents in 1994.

GOOD TO KNOW: Restrooms at various locations downtown including City Hall, the Central Library, Bookshop Santa Cruz, and parking garages.

START: Intersection of Mission Street, Front Street, and Pacific Avenue.

◆　**From the Town Clock cross Pacific Avenue and turn right.**

◆　**After passing 2019 North Pacific Avenue turn left and ascend the steep stairs.**

This staircase, built in 1920 and called the Anthony stairs, might get your heart pumping. It leads to School Street and the **Santa Cruz Mission State Historic Park**. The stairs are named after Elihu Anthony, one of the first Santa Cruz settlers who had a business on Pacific and a house at the top of the stairs which were wooden when first built. The steep stairway has seen a lot of drama over the years. [See "Fell over a bluff," below.]

◆　**From the top of the stairs**

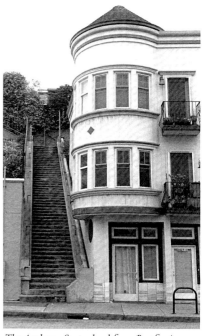

The Anthony Stairs lead from Pacific Avenue to School Street near the Santa Cruz Mission.

FELL OVER A BLUFF

Saturday noon G. M. Wolf of Ben Lomond left his wagon and two horses standing in front of M. Delaney's place on School Street. The horses ran away, and when the end of the street was reached they plunged against the plank railing, breaking it. The wagon and horses dropped several feet to the landing on the bluff, about five feet wide and covered with brush. One of the horses plunged over the bluff, fifty feet to the ground. The animal fell on its side. Spectators thought the animal was killed, but, to their surprise, the horse arose and walked away. With a block and tackle and ropes the wagon was raised to the sidewalk. The horse was also assisted to the sidewalk. Neither the wagon nor horses suffered any damage.

—*Santa Cruz Morning Sentinel*, December 10, 1899

proceed straight (west) on School Street. The building you are approaching to your left is an authentic adobe and the only part of the original mission remaining. It was built in the early 1800s.

◆ Turn left into the State Historic Park, if it is open, to see the 100-year old Avocado Tree, a picnic area, and a visitor center.

The actual mission itself (see marker in front of Holy Cross Church) is long gone. A reduced-scale replica of what the **mission chapel** might have looked like faces Mission Plaza. We pass the mission chapel on Walk 3.

◆ On the other side of School Street just past School Lane turn right at the cut-through behind the replica mission chapel before you get to Emmett Street. Walking activists worked hard to keep this cut-through open when the church tried to close this walkway.

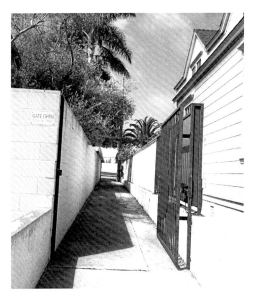

The pedestrian short cut behind the Mission was preserved by activists.

◆ Turn left on High Street where the walkway ends. You are now in front of Holy Cross Church built in 1889 on the site of an older mission chapel. Santa Cruz means "holy cross" in Spanish.

◆ Continue on High Street past Sylvar Street to where High Street ends at a cul-de-sac.

◆ Turn left and go up the ramp of the pedestrian bridge over Highway 1. When you descend on the other side of the highway you will still be on High Street which used to go through before this section of Highway 1 was made into a multilane highway segment.

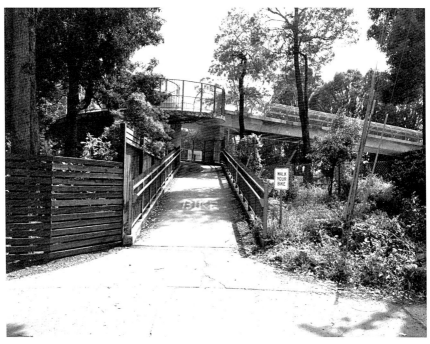

The pedestrian ramp over Highway 1 connects the two sections of High Street.

The cooperative condo building at 260 High Street is **Piedmont Court**, built in 1912. The Moorish style landmark has a central lobby and enclosed patio. Although not open to visitors, you can view the ornate interior in an online virtual tour, if available. The glass roof of the central patio came crashing down during the 1989 Loma Prieta earthquake.

◆   **After crossing Highland Avenue turn left and walk down Highland to Escalona Drive.**

◆   **Turn right on Escalona.** Across Highland hidden in the Vintage Faith Church is a coffee shop called The Abbey. There are many historic houses on Escalona Drive. Those interested in learning more can consult *The Sidewalk Companion to Santa Cruz Architecture*.

◆   **Cross Jordan Street and turn left.** You will pass the Georgiana Bruce Kirby house and historical plaque at 117 Jordan. Georgiana Bruce Kirby was an intellectual, author and feminist who believed in the equality of men and women. A local school is named after her.

◆ **Continue on Jordan Street to King Street.**

◆ **Cross King Street, turn right on King and walk to Walnut Avenue passing Mission Hill Middle School, built in 1931 as a junior high school** (Spanish Colonial Revival style).

◆ **Turn left on Walnut Avenue and walk to Mission Street.**

◆ **Cross Mission Street; continue on Walnut to Santa Cruz High School.**

This neo-classical high school designed by William Weeks celebrated its centennial in 2014. It was built to replace the wooden high school which burned on the site in 1913. The tall tree to the left of the front entrance is a Dawn Redwood. Unlike Coast Redwoods, Dawn Redwoods are deciduous. Their leaves turn orange in the fall before dropping. This species was thought to be extinct until it was discovered in China in 1941. Compare this tree with the Coast Redwoods you can see just downhill on Walnut Avenue past its junction with Lincoln Street.

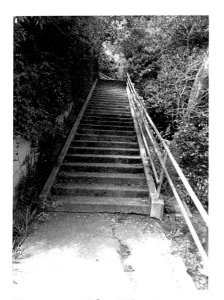

◆ **Continue downhill on Walnut going past the private "Pratchner" stairs on your left.**

◆ **Turn left to ascend the unlabeled stairs immediately down Walnut.** The contractors' names (Greenfield/ Costella) are stamped in the concrete below the first step. You ascend to Towne Terrace.

◆ **Follow Towne Terrace to Mission Street.**

These steps ascend from Walnut Avenue to Towne Terrace.

12

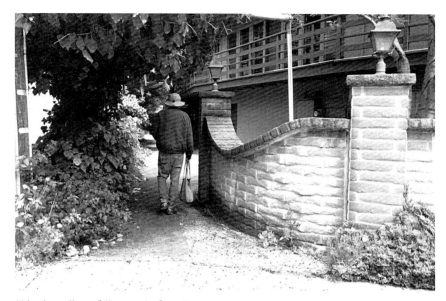

Take the walkway following the fence line behind the apartment building to Pine Place.

◆   **Turn right on Mission St.**

◆   **Turn right on Chrystal Terrace** (one block).

◆   **Turn left at the end of Chrystal Terrace. Take the walkway following the fence line behind the apartment building to Pine Place.** [See map and photo.]

◆   **Continue on Pine Place.** You will pass two 1937 International Style apartment houses on your right before reaching a paved path with a railing on your right.

◆   **Turn right on the Locust walkway and proceed downhill first on an asphalt path, then on stairs.** [See photo next page.] Enjoy the view of the white Hotel Palomar (also designed by William Weeks) adorned with the busts of conquistadors. The hotel built in 1928-29 survived the 1989 Loma Prieta earthquake which destroyed much of the Santa Cruz downtown.

◆   **Turn right at the bottom of the stairs and cross Chestnut**

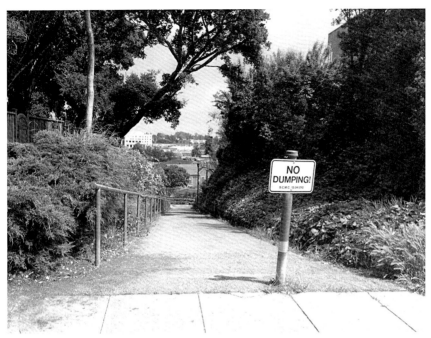

The Locust Street walkway is a shortcut from Mission Hill to downtown.

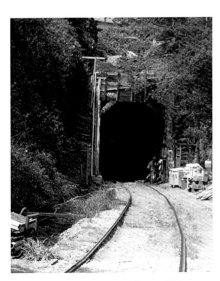

The railroad tunnel was built in 1875. We will see the other end of the tunnel on Walk 2.

at the marked crosswalk in front of the 1888 Stick-Eastlake Hinds House.

◆   **After crossing Chestnut Street turn left. Walk on Chestnut crossing Church Street and following Chestnut and the railroad tracks around the corner past Union Street.** On your left you will notice the railroad tunnel (built in 1875) under Mission Hill. If you look closely, you will see the steeple of Holy Cross Church on top of Mission Hill through the trees. During the summer and weekends much of the rest of the year the excursion train from Felton runs down the middle of Chestnut Street and through this tunnel on its way to and from the Boardwalk.

◆ **When safe, cross to the north side of Chestnut Street.**

◆ **Turn left on Center Street and walk to the intersection of Center and Mission Streets.**

◆ **Cross Center Street at the traffic signal.**

◆ **Cross Mission Street.**

◆ **Turn right and cross Pacific Avenue back to** START **at the Town Clock.**

Reference:

Chase, John Leighton and Gregory, Daniel P., *The Sidewalk Companion to Santa Cruz Architecture*, Third edition, edited by Judith Steen, The Museum of Art & History, 2005.

BUS ACCESS TO WALK STARTS

The METRO bus system provides a good way to get to the walks in this book without a car. Bus schedules are available at www.scmtd.com. All of the walks are near bus stops.

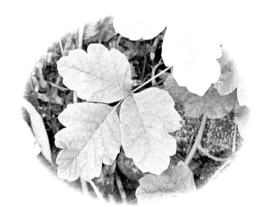

Poison Oak

2 CITY HALL— POGONIP LOOP

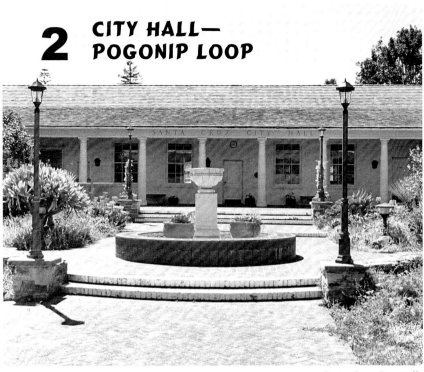

Santa Cruz City Hall

6.3 miles / 650 feet elevation gain

WALK SUMMARY

This walk takes you from the heart of downtown Santa Cruz past historic sites to one of the city open space parks. It is one of the more strenuous walks in this book.

GOOD TO KNOW: Restrooms at City Hall from courtyard across from Council Chambers.

START: Santa Cruz City Hall, on the corner of Center and Church Streets. Enter the courtyard from Center Street.

Visitors from out of town are often surprised at the Santa Cruz City Hall building. They have told me they were expecting a larger building instead of the 1937-38 single story Monterey Colonial Revival building with its columned galleria. Be sure to check out the inner courtyard with its

17

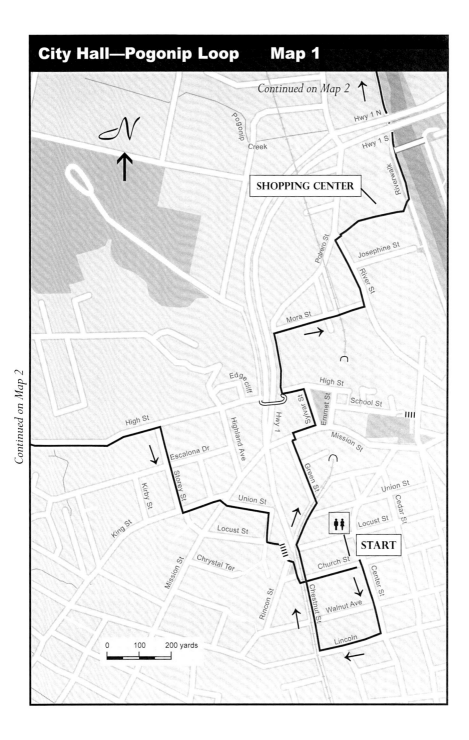

Continued on Map 2

Continued on Map 2

SHOPPING CENTER

START

0   100   200 yards

fountains between City Hall and the two-story annex on Church Street. The rose garden on the Locust Street side of the building is a special treat for rose aficionados.

The unusual Kapok Tree (Floss Silk Tree) by the rose garden entrance on the Center Street side of the building is a sight to see. This South American native is easily identifiable by its trunk covered with thorns. In spring it sports showy pink-red flowers; in fall it rains fluffy fibers which the U.S. Navy has used to stuff life jackets.

◆   **From the front of City Hall on Center Street cross Church Street and walk past the Civic Auditorium to Lincoln Street** [see map]. As you pass Fire Station Number 1 notice the plaque honoring early volunteer firefighters.

Across the street at Center and Lincoln is the Calvary Episcopal Church (1864), the oldest church building in Santa Cruz and site of the Penny University, a long-running salon which meets weekly for discussions.

◆   **Turn right on Lincoln Street.** The ca.1894 row houses on the corner of Lincoln and Chestnut were saved from the wrecking ball in 1973 by Chuck and Esther Abbott, after whom Abbott Square is named. They also financed the Mark Abbott Memorial Lighthouse on West Cliff Drive in memory of their son who died in a surfing accident.

◆   **Turn right on Chestnut Street.**

◆   **Walk up Chestnut following the train tracks.** The two-story building across the street at the corner of Walnut Avenue and Chestnut is

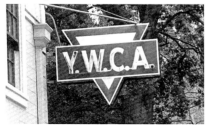

The Walnut Avenue Women's Center still displays the historic YWCA sign.

the 1927 YWCA building (the old sign is on the Walnut Avenue side of the building). It is now a non-profit Women's Center. The tree near the front door on Chestnut is a Ginkgo, native to China. This species is the only plant to survive from the age of the dinosaurs. Its fan-shaped leaves make it easy to identify.

After you cross Walnut Avenue you can see several large Coast Redwood trees abutting the sidewalk. These redwoods provide a good comparison to the Dawn Redwood further up the hill in front of Santa Cruz High School. The Coast Redwood is the California state tree.

Across the street at the corner of Walnut Avenue and Chestnut Street is another large tree, a Bunya Bunya, a conifer native to Australia. These trees produce 10-pound female cones which can cause serious damage when they fall. Bunya Bunya trees were popular landscaping trees in the 1800s. The house behind the tree was built in 1888.

◆ **Turn left on Green Street after Chestnut Street curves** and proceed up the steep hill past more historic houses. Green Street is one way going downhill, but not for us. What do you suppose the granite block next to the street at 127 Green was for? Might it have helped you step up into a horse-drawn carriage in 1870?

Notice too, the granite curbstones as you near the top of the hill. At the corner of Green and Mission Streets is a marker noting the site of the first Protestant church in Santa Cruz (1848-50).

◆ **Wave politely to catch drivers' eyes as you cross Mission Street** in the painted crosswalk.

◆ **Turn right on Mission Street** once you have crossed.

◆ **Turn Left on Sylvar Street.** The house at 109 Sylvar is the oldest frame house in Santa Cruz, built about 1850. Here lived Francisco Alzina, first sheriff after California became a state. Alzina stowed away on the USS Constitution when it was in Barcelona Harbor and came to the U.S.

◆ **At the end of Sylvar turn left on High Street.**

◆ **Turn right on the paved path at the end of High Street.** Follow this path down the hill to unsigned Mora Street.

◆ **Turn right on Mora Street** and walk down the hill to River Street. As you cross the railroad tracks look to your right to catch a glimpse of the northern end of the railroad tunnel under Mission Hill visible on Walk 1.

Near where you are standing just west of the San Lorenzo River was the site of the first mission built in 1791. It was moved to the top of Mission Hill by 1794 to escape flooding. You can see Holy Cross Church at the top of the hill if you take a few steps to your right toward the garden store.

◆ **Turn left on River Street.**

◆ **Cross River Street at the traffic signal at Potrero Street.**

◆ **Follow the sidewalk past the stores to the levee.**

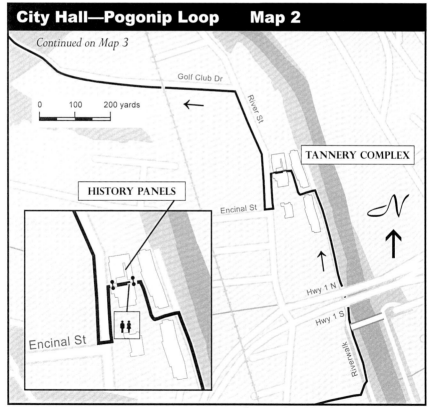

Continued on Map 3

Continued on Map 1

◆   **Ascend the levee path heading to your left.**

◆   **Follow the levee path** UNDER **the highway** once you have passed the bicycle/pedestrian bridge over the river. Just after passing under the highway you will cross a short bridge over Pogonip Creek as it flows into the San Lorenzo River. Later on this hike you will see this same creek in a woodland setting.

The vista opens up a bit, and riparian habitat is to your right along the river bank. Ahead you can see the barn red buildings of the Tannery Arts Center. This complex of 100 affordable live/work units and art studios was built on the site of the historic Salz Tannery.

There is lots to explore at the Tannery Complex including a café, a theater, history panels, and numerous art installations. Periodically there are festivals and studio tours.

My favorite are the sliding panels depicting the history of the tannery itself. Large photographs, many by Ansel Adams, show the tanning process and the craftsmen who cured and finished the leather.

◆   As you approach the complex **take the right fork of the trail** and walk behind the apartments. [See photo below.]

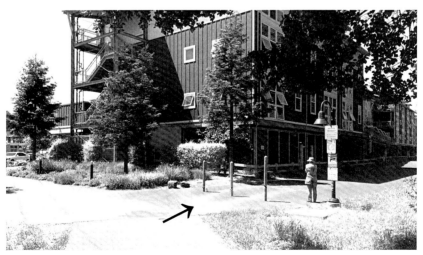

Take the right fork of the path as you approach the Tannery Complex.

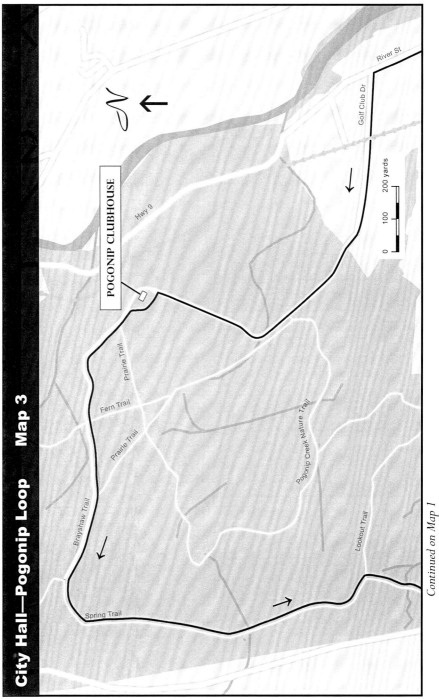

City Hall—Pogonip Loop   Map 3

POGONIP CLUBHOUSE

Hwy 9

River St

Golf Club Dr

0   100   200 yards

Prairie Trail

Fern Trail

Prairie Trail

Brayshaw Trail

Pogonip Creek Nature Trail

Lookout Trail

Spring Trail

Continued on Map 1

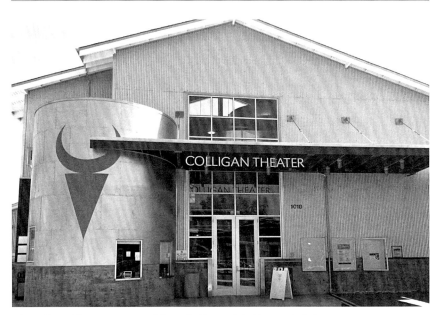

The Colligan Theater was created from the former Salz Tannery hide house.

◆ After passing the first building, turn left to reach the large courtyard where you can see the Colligan Theater and several sculptures.

◆ Continue in an upriver direction past the Radius Gallery and through a passageway on your left into another courtyard with a café and the history panels. [See inset on map 2.]

◆ Walk to River Street through an opening opposite the cafe.

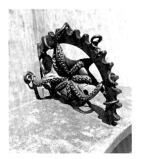

◆ Walk left along the sidewalk to the traffic signal and cross River Street.

EARLY RETURN

If you are ready to return to START, turn left instead of right on River Street after crossing Hwy. 9 and walk on River Street back to downtown.

Bench detail from the Tannery courtyard.

◆　**Turn right on the other side of River Street and walk to Golf Club Drive.**

◆　**Turn left on Golf Club Drive** passing under the railroad bridge soon arriving at the entrance to the Pogonip, a 640 acre city greenbelt property. The name "Pogonip" refers to a cold winter fog. The almost wilderness quality of this city greenbelt is partially derived from the fact that it abuts Henry Cowell State Park and open space areas on the UCSC campus making for a large undeveloped area which supports many plant and animal species.

◆　**Follow Golf Club Drive up the hill** eventually arriving at the unrestored Pogonip Clubhouse. Behind you as you climb are expansive views of Santa Cruz and the Monterey Bay including the Tannery buildings you have just visited.

At the top of Golf Club Drive is the Craftsman-style Pogonip Clubhouse which began as a golf playground in 1911 and developed into a polo club in the 1930s. The polo club was unique in featuring women teams as well as mixed men/women teams. An interpretive sign provides some very interesting details. Dorothy Deming Wheeler, whose childhood home on Beach Hill we see on Walk 8 was the prime mover in establishing a polo field at Pogonip. Fred Swanton was the main promoter and planner for the earlier golf club. You can see Fred Swanton's home on Walk 5.

◆　**Take the left fork to see the front of the Clubhouse.** The meadow in front of the building once contained a putting green. Around the side of the building one can see the filled-in swimming pool and the remains of the tennis courts.

◆　**Continue past the**

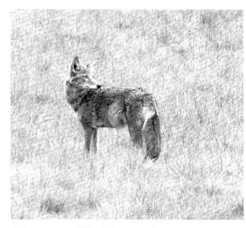

Perhaps you will be lucky enough to see a coyote at the Pogonip.

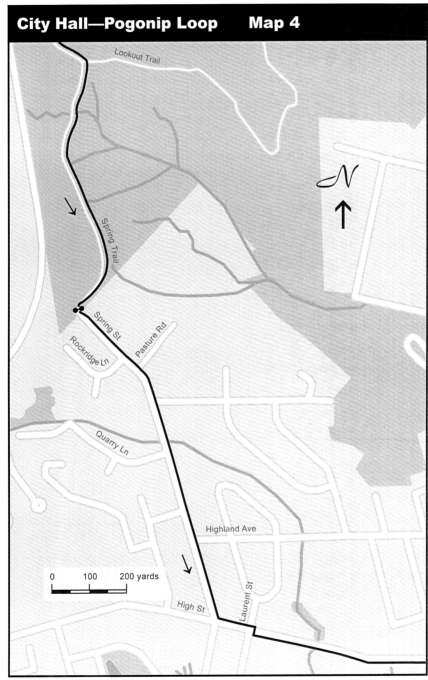

Lookout Trail

Spring Trail

Spring St

Rockridge Ln

Pasture Rd

Quarry Ln

Highland Ave

0   100   200 yards

High St

Laurent St

continued on Map 1.

Clubhouse to the marked Brayshaw Trail which continues up the hill past the Prairie Trail, the Fern Trail and the fenced-off cistern on your left.

The trail steepens just before you join the Spring Trail.

Soon one is transported to a natural wonderland with a variety of habitats including mixed evergreen forest with Coast Live Oaks and Bay Laurels, second growth Redwood forest, and meadows. Here are the sounds of water flowing, birds calling, and the wind in the treetops. You might even be lucky enough to see a deer or coyote.

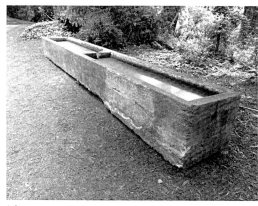

This concrete watering trough was used when the Pogonip was part of the Cowell Ranch.

◆ **Turn left on the Spring Trail.** Soon the sound of Pogonip Creek fills the air. A concrete watering trough once serviced oxen and horses. Look for large yellow banana slugs in this damp area of the redwood forest.

Your path gradually takes you out of the forest and into a meadow with more fantastic views.

◆ **Continue on the Spring Trail past the Lookout Trail to Spring Street.**

◆ **Turn left on Spring Street and walk to High Street.**

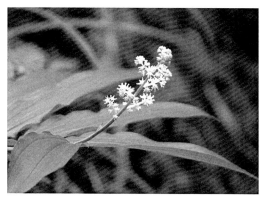

Fat Solomons Seal blooms at Pogonip in the spring.

BANANA SLUGS

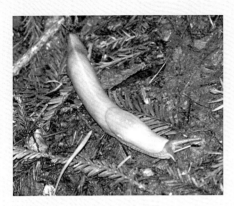

Most active during moist, cool times these mollusks excrete slime to keep themselves from drying out. They eat organic matter and enrich the soil. They are the mascot of UC Santa Cruz.

◆ **Turn left on High Street.**

◆ **Cross High at Laurent Street.**

◆ **Continue on High Street to Storey Street.**

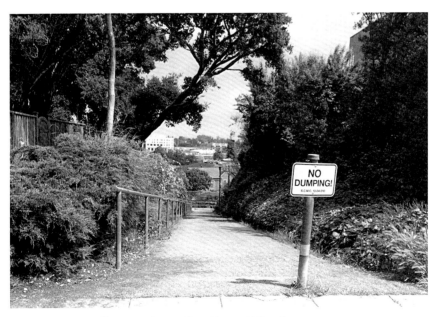

The Locust Street walkway is a shortcut from Mission Hill to downtown.

◆ **Turn right on Storey Street and walk to King Street.**

◆ **Cross King and turn left. Walk to Mission Street.**

◆ **Cross Mission Street.**

◆ **Continue straight on Union Street.**

◆ **At the end of Union turn right on Pine Place.** This street is one way, but we can turn right—an advantage of walking! On your left the house at 410 once belonged to Lucy Ann Field Wanzer, M.D. who was the first woman to earn a medical degree from a California school in 1876.

◆ **Turn left on the asphalt Locust Street path** leading downhill. From our vantage point we can see the solar panels shading the City Hall parking lot.

◆ **Turn right at the bottom of the stairs and cross Chestnut at the marked crosswalk** waving politely at drivers to encourage them to obey traffic laws and yield to pedestrians as you use the crosswalk.

◆ **Walk down Church Street.** Just after you pass the very large redwood at 333 Church Street, there is an interpretive panel explaining how "Solar Energy Powers City Hall."

Back to START

References:

Chase, John Leighton and Gregory, Daniel P., *The Sidewalk Companion to Santa Cruz Architecture*, Third edition, Edited by Judith Steen, The Museum of Art & History, 2005.

Ritter, Matt, *A California Guide to the Trees Among Us*, Hayday, 2011.

Martin, Joan Gilbert & McInerney-Meagher, Colleen, *Pogonip, Jewel of Santa Cruz*, Otter B Books, 2007.

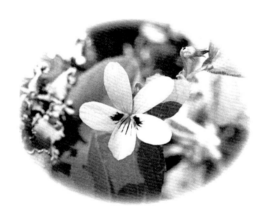

Two-eyed violet

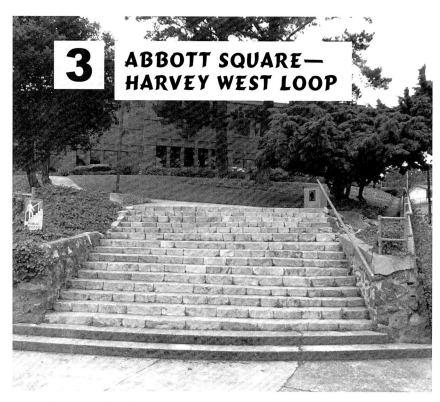

3 ABBOTT SQUARE— HARVEY WEST LOOP

3.5 miles / 500 feet elevation gain

WALK SUMMARY

W e start this loop at Abbott Square, an often bustling plaza nestled between the Museum of Art and History (MAH) and buildings on Pacific Avenue. Here we can find food, often music or events, and restrooms. The MAH itself is worth a visit.

Forming part of the Square enclosure is the Octagon, the 1882 Hall of Records at 118 Cooper Street. Cooper Street was named after the Cooper family who settled in Santa Cruz in the 1850s and who were related to the author James Fenimore Cooper.

GOOD TO KNOW: This walk may be strenuous for some. There are multiple stairways. Restrooms at start and at Harvey West Park.

START: Abbott Square, downtown Santa Cruz.

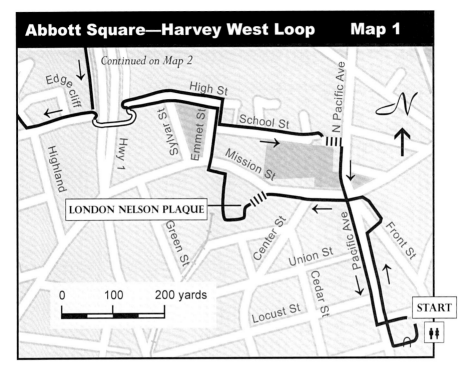

◆ **From Abbott Square exit to Pacific Avenue through the arched tunnel opposite the food area.**

◆ **Turn right on Pacific** passing a slim columnar monument in memory of the seven people who lost their lives in the 1989 Loma Prieta earthquake which destroyed much of the downtown.

A local favorite is the bronze statue of Tom Scribner by Marghc McMahon. Scribner was an iconic figure in the 1970s playing his musical saw in front of the Saint George Hotel. A World War I veteran, Scribner had been a lumberjack, labor organizer and member of the Communist Party.

◆ **Continue on Pacific Avenue to the World War I Memorial.**

◆ **Turn right and cross Front Street to the Post Office** which is on the National Register of Historic Places. Inside the 1911 building are several 1936 murals celebrating local agriculture and industry painted by Carmel artist Henrietta Shore as part of the WPA (Works Progress Administration) program, a Federal program which provided jobs during the Great Depression. Shore was influenced by Mexican muralists Diego Rivera and Jose Clemente Orozco. A modest wall display gives information on Shore's life as well as on the historic building. Additionally, above the post office boxes are historical photos of the building's construction in 1911 including a fascinating architectual drawing.

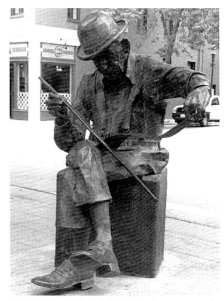

◆ **Turn left on Front Street** (or right if you are exiting the Post Office) and walk to the corner of Front/Pacific/Mission Streets.

Tom Scribner played the musical saw on Pacific Avenue in the 1970s.

The short pillars and sidewalk compass at this corner honor Santa Cruz's sister cities: Shingu, Japan; Jinotepe, Nicaragua; Puerto La Cruz, Venezuela; Sestri Levante, Italy; and Alushta, Ukraine.

◆ **Cross Front Street/Pacific Avenue and walk up Mission Street past Center Street.** Across the street you can see the mosaic mural created by art teacher Kathleen Crocetti and her Mission Hill Middle School students and community volunteers in 2016 to commemorate the 25th anniversary of the Santa Cruz Mission State Historic Park.

◆ **Ascend the granite stairs on your left.** These steps (shown in the title picture for this walk) and the adjoining wall next to the sidewalk going up the hill are all that remain of the Mission Hill Grammar School built in 1879. At the top of the stairs is a monument to "Louden" [London] Nelson, a former enslaved black man, who came to California with his master Matthew Nelson in 1849 during the gold rush and subsequently obtained his freedom. Because he never learned to read and write, he knew the value of an education. At his death in 1860, London Nelson willed the property he had acquired to the Santa Cruz School District "for the purpose of promoting the interest in education." The silhouette on the monument represents Nelson since no record of his appearance exists. Nelson's first name was London, but he is memorialized as Louden by poor penmanship on the part of record keepers.

◆ **Take the path leading to your left going around the side of the brick building.** You will pass a locked staircase leading down to Chestnut Street. (That section of Chestnut was once named Cherry.) The city allowed this staircase to be locked to the public in 2013 because of neglect by the property owner and abuse by some members of the public. Historically these stairs have been an important pedestrian shortcut between Mission and Chestnut Streets. Without proper commitment, oversight and stewardship by the city, other historic pedestrian shortcuts could be lost to the community.

◆ **Go through the parking area and return to Mission Street.** Across Mission in a break in the 1884 historic stone wall one can see steps leading up to a dead end at the fenced playground of Holy Cross School. These once led to the first Holy Cross School of the 1860s.

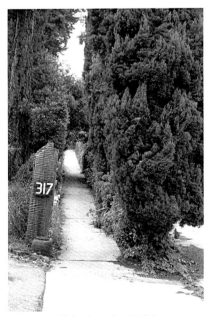

This sidewalk leads to the 1910 Logan stairway.

◆ **Cross Mission Street at Emmet Street.**

◆ **Walk past the Mission replica** (or stop in for a tour if you are so inclined).

◆ **Turn left on High Street and continue to what appears to be the end of High Street.**

◆ **From the cul-de-sac go up the ramp of the pedestrian bridge over Highway 1.** When you descend on the other side

34

Abbott Square—Harvey West Loop   Map 2

HARVEY WEST PARK

Meadow Rd   Meadow Ct

Evergreen St

Coral St

Meadow Rd

Sheldon Ave

Bolla Row

Highland Ct

Highland Avenue

Hillcrest Ter

Edge Cliff

High St

0   100   200 yards

Continued on Map 1

of the bridge you will still be on High Street which used to go through before the highway was made into a multi-lane freeway segment.

◆ **Circle around to the north side of High Street and continue to Highland Avenue.**

◆ **Cross Highland Avenue and turn right.**

◆ **Stay on the sidewalk on Highland.** The sidewalk continues up the hill and passes between two driveways to a 1910 concrete staircase (Logan Stairs).

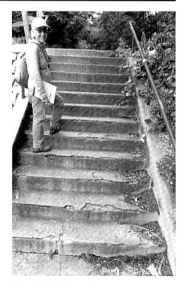

The 1910 Logan Stairs.

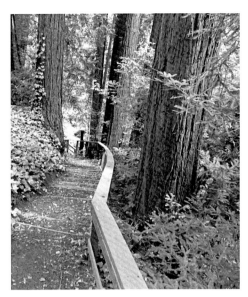

[See photo.] This staircase reputedly once led to the estate of Judge James Logan who developed the loganberry. The stairway cuts across the base of the hairpin curve which Highland Avenue makes as it climbs up the hill. Logan's house was demolished in 1948 and the estate turned into a subdivision.

◆ **Continue straight at the top of the stairs, continuing on Highland.** There is no sidewalk on this part of Highland Avenue. Walk with care on the left facing oncoming traffic. Soon the sidewalk resumes.

The path from Meadow Court to Harvey West Park includes several stairways through the redwood forest.

◆ **Turn right at Sheldon Avenue and cross Highland Avenue.**

◆ **Continue on Sheldon Avenue.**

◆ **Turn right on Meadow Road.**

◆ **Continue straight on unsigned Meadow Court. Do not follow Meadow Road when it curves to the left.** [See Map 2.]

◆ **At the end of Meadow Court turn right to the staircase.**

◆ **Descend the stairs and cross over a short bridge keeping straight. Stay on the main trail. Turn left at forks.** There are several informal use trails. Keep an eye out for poison oak. You will eventually emerge in the main part of Harvey West Park which hosts numerous recreational facilities as well as welcome restrooms.

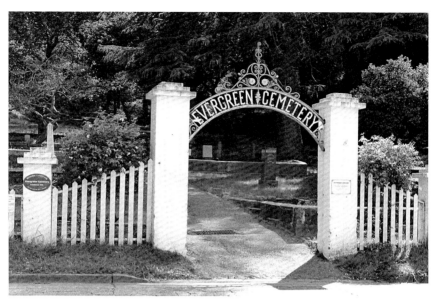

Many early settlers of Santa Cruz are buried in Evergreen Cemetery.

The entire trail from Meadow Court to the lower part of Harvey West Park goes for about 0.4 of a mile through a dappled redwood forest, down multiple sets of stairs and switchbacks. You might hear the sounds of baseball games far below. In the spring the forest is dotted with pink and white California Hedge-nettle, blue-flowered Western Hound's Tongue, Violets and other flowers. Take care not to step on yellow banana slugs, artfully disguised as fallen Bay Laurel leaves.

◆   **Continue straight at the switchback about halfway down the grade.** Just beyond the switchback there is a large multi-trunked California Bay Laurel Tree. This native tree has aromatic leaves. You will eventually emerge at a T intersection by a split rail fence and a bicycle pump track.

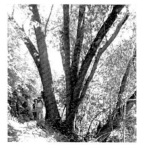

◆   **Turn right at the T intersection and continue on the trail to the train engine behind another fence.** This is Southern Pacific 1298, a small switcher engine built in 1917.

California Bay Laurel just beyond the switchback.

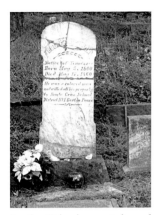

London Nelson's grave is located near the Chinese section of Evergreen Cemetery.

Children were once allowed to climb on this oil-powered steam engine.

◆ **Proceed from the park to Evergreen Street.** On the way you pass by the group picnic areas and some truly massive Coast Live Oaks. [See the photo on p. 40.]

◆ **Continue on Evergreen Street to Evergreen Cemetery enclosed behind a white picket fence on your right.** Here are buried many Santa Cruz pioneers including Civil War veterans, Chinese immigrants, and London [Louden] Nelson who gave his property to the school district. Although his name was London, the name "Louden" persists on his gravestone and the monument we saw on Mission Hill. Nelson's grave is up the hill on the left as you look from the street near the Chinese section of the cemetery.

The oldest grave is that of 19-day-old Julia Arcan who died on July 19, 1850. Julia's mother, Abigail, was pregnant when she and her family were stranded in Death Valley during the winter of 1849-50. Abigail is said to have named Death Valley. Julia's grave can be seen from the street on the right side near a telephone pole.

◆ **Once you leave Evergreen Cemetery, continue on Evergreen Street to where it meets Coral Street.**

◆ **Take the paved path leading up the hill from Coral Street** [See photo next page].KEEP RIGHT AND WATCH OUT for fast downhill bicyclists. If you are walking in May, the California Buckeye will be in full bloom. These native trees often lose their leaves during the summer but in spring explode like the Fourth of July with white flower spikes. In fall you might be lucky enough to find some smooth brown buckeyes on the ground about the size of walnuts.

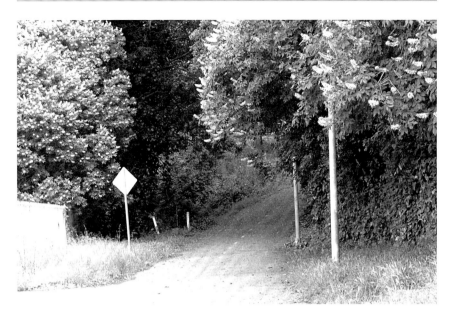

In May the multi-use path from Evergreen Street to High Street is bordered by California Buckeyes in glorious bloom.

◆   **The path ends at the High Street pedestrian overpass** over Hwy 1.

◆   **Turn left to walk over the pedestrian bridge back to Mission Plaza**, the park in front of Holy Cross Church and the Mission Replica.

◆   **Turn right on Emmet Street.**

◆   **Turn left on School Street.**

◆   **Descend the steep steps [Anthony Stairs] at the end of School Street.** Partway down the stairs is the site for the obligatory photo of City Council candidates for their campaign brochures. It's a grand view of the city.

◆   **Turn right on Pacific Avenue, cross Mission Street and walk to Cooper Street.**

◆   **Turn left on Cooper and return to** START.

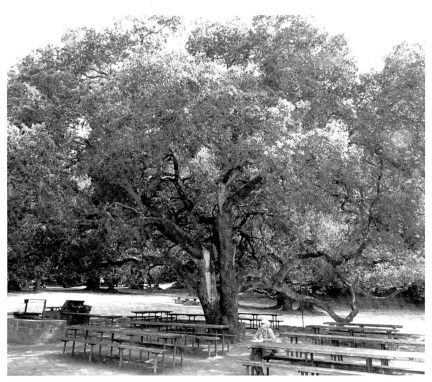

COAST LIVE OAK

This magnificent evergreen oak is native to California and grows, as one would guess from its name, along the California coast from about Mendocino to Baja. It is the eponymous tree after which Oakland and Live Oak (in Santa Cruz County) are named.

References:

Ritter, Matt, *A California Guide to the Trees Among Us*. Hayday, 2011.

Martin, Joan Gilbert and McInerney-Meagher, Coleen, *Pogonip, Jewel of Santa Cruz*, Otter B Books, 2007.

Rogers, Paul. "Santa Cruz pays tribute to street musician," *San Jose Mercury News.* 1993-06-24. SCPL Local History.

Johnson, LeRoy and Jean, *Julia, Death Valley's Youngest Victim,* Second Edition, 1996.

Muth, Deborah, *Santa Cruz Through Time,* America Through Time, 2019.

A DEATH VALLEY RESCUE

William Lewis Manley, who with John Rogers found a way out of Death Valley and came back with provisions to rescue the Bennett and Arcan families, wrote an account of the rescue that was published in 1894. The book, *Death Valley in '49*, describes the 250-mile escape. There were four young children in the Bennett/Arcan party.

Parents John-Baptiste and Abigail Arcan with two-year-old Charlie eventually settled in Santa Cruz. What is not mentioned in the book is that Abigail was pregnant with Julia (later born in Santa Cruz) during the ordeal.

In Manley's words:

"Bennett and Arcane assisted their wives down along the little narrow ledge . . . , keeping their faces toward the rocky wall, and feeling carefully for every footstep." p 221

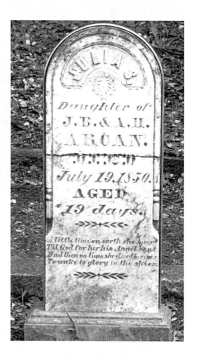

"There was a little water left in the canteens of Bennett and Arcane, to be given only to the children, who would cry when thirsty. . . ." p. 223

"We were slowly leaving Death Valley behind us with its sad memories and sufferings. We were leaving behind the dead bodies of several who had traveled with us and been just as strong and hopeful as we. We had left behind us all in our possession in that terrible spot. . . ." p. 238

Reference:

Manley, William Lewis, *Death Valley in '49*, The Pacific Tree and Vine Co., San Jose, CA, 1894.

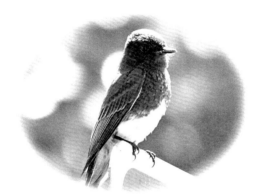

Black Phoebe

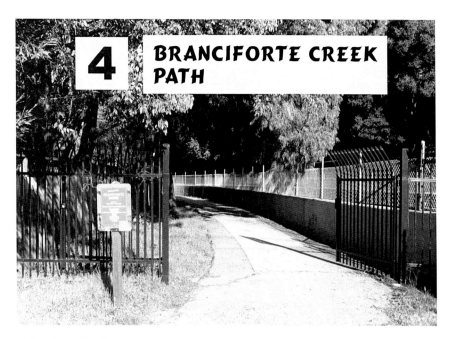

BRANCIFORTE CREEK PATH

3.5 miles / 50 feet elevation gain

WALK SUMMARY

On this walk starting in downtown Santa Cruz we follow one of the tributaries of the San Lorenzo River upstream from its channelized junction with the river to the more natural riparian reaches.

GOOD TO KNOW: There are restrooms at Abbott Square, San Lorenzo Park, and Grant Park. Sections of this walk are on dirt paths which can be muddy after a rain. Sections of this walk are closed at night.

START: Abbott Square

◆ **From Abbott Square exit to Cooper Street.**

◆ **Turn right on Cooper.** The Leonard Building across the street was built in 1894 and survived the 1989 Loma Prieta earthquake. If you want to verify which way is north, check out its weather vane.

◆ **Cross Front Street and continue straight** on a passageway between a restaurant on your left and an office building on your right. [See

43

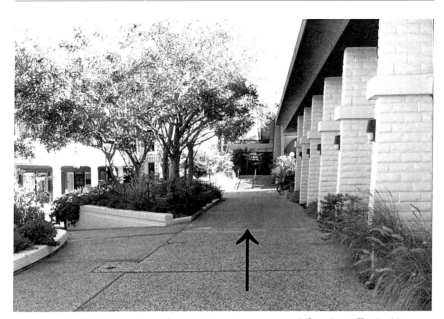

Continue straight on a passageway between a restaurant on your left and an office building on your right to the Chinatown Bridge across Front Street.

photo above.] This area between the San Lorenzo River and the downtown once housed the last (of four) Chinatowns in Santa Cruz. It was destroyed in the devastating December 1955 flood and its population dispersed. Ahead the Chinese Gate at the entrance to the pedestrian bridge over the San Lorenzo River commemorates the last Santa Cruz Chinatown.

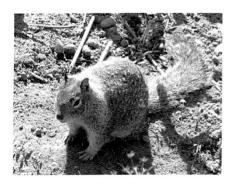

California Ground Squirrels are common along the banks of the San Lorenzo River.

◆ **Continue straight to unsigned River Street and cross to the foot bridge.**

◆ **Cross the San Lorenzo River on the Chinatown pedestrian bridge straight ahead.** Take a minute to pause on the bridge to look for bird and animal life both in the river and on its banks. California Ground Squirrels abound.

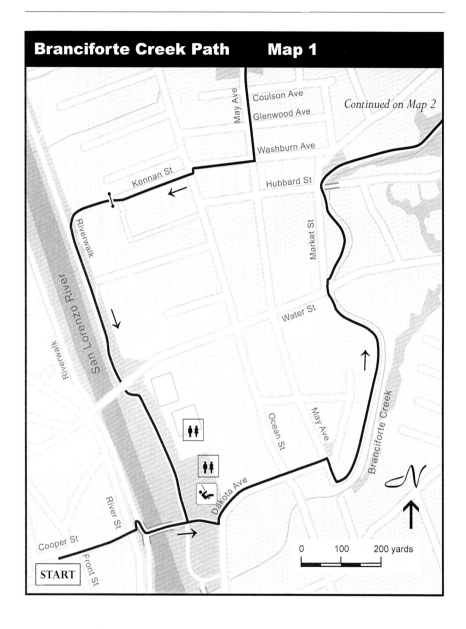

Branciforte Creek Path   Map 1

Coulson Ave
May Ave
Glenwood Ave
Continued on Map 2

Washburn Ave

Kennan St
Hubbard St

Riverwalk

Market St

San Lorenzo River

Water St

Riverwalk

Ocean St
May Ave
Branciforte Creek

Dakota Ave

River St

Cooper St

Front St

START

0   100   200 yards

Once across the bridge we are in San Lorenzo Park. This park and the lands surrounding it are the only part of the lower San Lorenzo River that is not constrained behind levees which were built by the Army Corps of Engineers after the 1955 flood.

Chinatown was not the only area flooded in the Christmas 1955 deluge. People, cars, and houses all over downtown were swept away; rescuers plied downtown streets in rowboats in darkness as electricity and phone lines were down.

◆ **Walk on the path to Dakota Avenue from the Chinatown Bridge passing the duck pond on your left.** At the junction of Dakota Avenue and the park path is a plaque marking the location of Bull and Bear fights in early Santa Cruz until outlawed in 1867.

My favorite part of the park is the grove of Cork Oak trees along Dakota Street. I love the spongy bark of these trees which looks just like (surprise!) the wine corks which are produced from it. Every time I walk past these trees, I think of Ferdinand the Bull from the Monro Leaf picture book of my childhood.

◆ **Turn left on Dakota Avenue and walk to Ocean Street.**

◆ **Cross Ocean Street at the flashing beacon and continue straight on Dakota.**

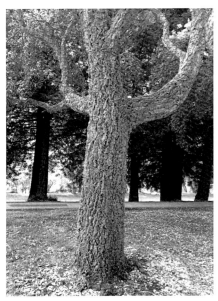

◆ **Turn right on May Avenue** and continue to where it ends at Branciforte Creek. There used to be a foot bridge across the creek here but it had to be taken out due to damage from the 1955 flood.

◆ **Turn left on the Branciforte Creek Path.** This path (and the one on the opposite side of the creek) were originally built as access roads for maintenance of the now channelized Branciforte Creek. The levee and channelization projects were completed in 1959

A cork oak in San Lorenzo Park.

as part of flood control to "prevent Branciforte Creek from repeating some of its past winter escapades" as the *Santa Cruz Sentinel* phrased it. (*Santa Cruz Sentinel*, September 11, 1958.)

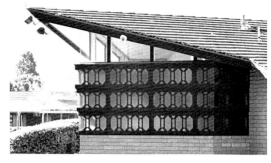

The Water Street Medical Plaza was designed in 1964 by Aaron Green.

The path, which is closed at night, provides a leafy respite to busy Ocean Street. Amazingly the tall trees lining the way still provide some habitat despite the tons of concrete encasing the creek bed. When scouting this walk, we saw a Red-shouldered Hawk in a tree top as we walked along.

The path leaves the creek at the Water Street Medical Plaza. This medical office complex was designed in 1964 by Aaron Green who had worked in Frank Lloyd Wright's studio.

◆ **Wend your way through the parking lot to Water Street.**

◆ **Cross Water Street at the traffic signal.**

◆ **Cross Market Street.**

◆ **A few feet up Market Street turn right onto the continuation of the Branciforte Creek path.**

◆ **Go around the pedestrian bridge over the creek at Hubbard Street by turning right on Market and immediately right again to get back on the creek path.** [See photo p. 48.]

◆ **Continue alongside the channelized creek for less than half a mile to where the concrete walls end.** The whole creek miraculously comes alive with vegetation cascading down the banks. The view of the creek improves greatly now there are no concrete walls; you can hear its gurgles, and wildlife is more abundant. What a difference!

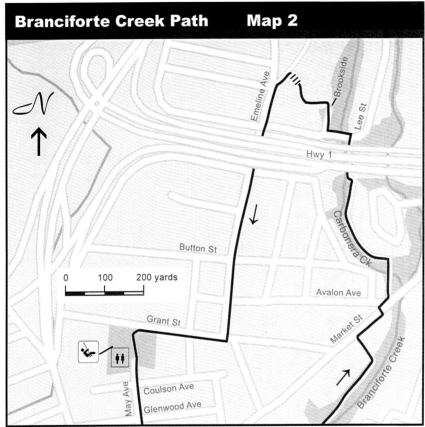

Branciforte Creek Path   Map 2

Emeline Ave

Brookside

Lee St

Hwy 1

Carbonera Ck

Button St

0   100   200 yards

Avalon Ave

Grant St

Market St

Coulson Ave

May Ave

Glenwood Ave

Branciforte Creek

Continued on Map 1

California Buckeyes put on quite a show when they are in bloom in May in this section of the creek. This native tree grows only in California. During the late summer through winter they lose their leaves and are bare, but when they bloom they resemble firecrackers going off.

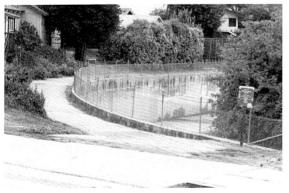

Continuation of the Branciforte path after Hubbard Street.

48

◆   **Soon the path ends at Market Street again.**

◆   **Turn right and walk about 200 feet to the unmarked pedestrian crossing of Market Street at Avalon Avenue** indicated by the yellow access ramp in the sidewalk.

◆   **Cross Market Street here being careful of speeding drivers** who might be less aware of pedestrians since this legal crosswalk is not marked with paint to alert drivers.

◆   **Cross Avalon Avenue in the marked crosswalk and continue a few feet up Market Street.**

◆   **Bear left on the paved creekside path.** As you cross the next pedestrian bridge, you overlook Carbonera Creek which joins Branciforte Creek near Market Street.

◆   **Turn left** IMMEDIATELY **after crossing the pedestrian bridge.** Do not be deterred by the NO TRESPASSING sign. This dirt path is open to the public. The NO TRESPASSING sign refers to the private property next

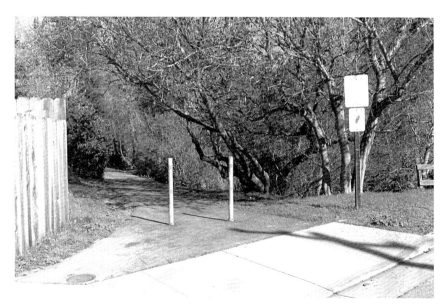

After crossing Avalon Avenue bear left on the paved creekside path.

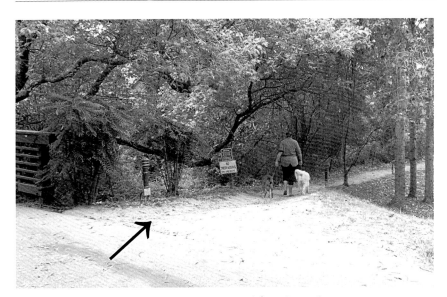

Immediately after crossing the pedestrian bridge turn left on this trail.

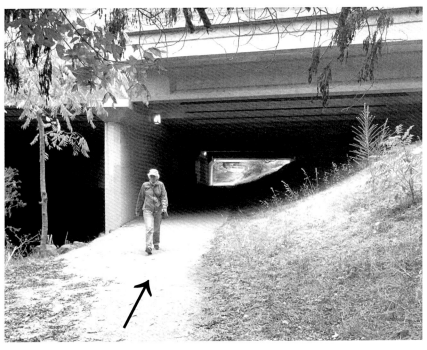

Walk under the Highway 1 bridge to Lee Street.

to the path. Please respect the neighbors and stay on the path. [See photo on the previous page.]

◆   **Follow the path behind the townhouses, continuing straight on the left fork when it divides.**

◆   **Walk under the Highway 1 bridge to Lee Street.**

◆   **Cross Lee to the sidewalk and turn left.** The street bridge gives you a good opportunity to look upstream on Carbonera Creek.

◆   **Turn right on Brookside Avenue.**

◆   **Walk to the end of Brookside and continue past the cul-de-sac to the parking lot.** You are now on the extensive grounds of the Santa Cruz County Health Department. This complex of buildings grew from the "County Poor Farm" built in 1877 to care for sick indigent men to a 1925 hospital which until 1933 was the only general hospital in North Santa Cruz County. Today there is no inpatient hospital here. The campus currently houses a variety of health care clinics, human services and health services including the Community Traffic Safety Coalition staff.

◆   **Turn immediately left once you are in the parking lot and walk behind a building to another parking area.**

◆   **Climb the wooden stairway on your right across the parking area.**

◆   **Turn left at the top of the stairs and walk on the asphalt sidewalk to Emeline Avenue.**

◆   **Turn left on Emeline.**

◆   **Continue on Emeline under the Highway 1 bridge,** this time on a sidewalk instead of on a creek path.

◆   **Cross Grant Street where Emeline ends.**

◆   **Turn right on Grant and walk to the entrance of Grant Park.**

◆   **Walk through the park past the restroom and exit out the back gate on May Avenue.**

◆   **Cross Washburn Avenue at the stop sign and turn right on Washburn.**

◆   **Walk to Ocean Street.**

◆   **Cross Ocean Street to Kennan Street at the traffic signal.**

◆   **Walk to the end of Kennan Street. At the end of Kennan there is a gate. Pass through the gate.** Sometimes one has to PULL HARD **to open the gate** which tends to stick.

◆   **Pass through the gate and follow the walkway to the river**

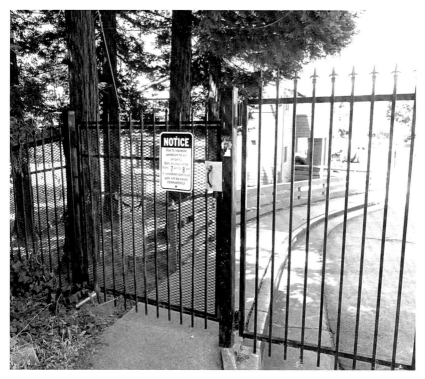

Sometimes the Kennan Street gate tends to stick. You may need to pull hard.

levee straight ahead.

◆   **Follow the asphalt path up to the Riverwalk.**

◆   **Turn left on the Riverwalk, and return to the pedestrian bridge near the County Building at San Lorenzo Park.** You will pass under the Water Street bridge on the way.

◆   **Turn right to cross the San Lorenzo River on the Chinatown pedestrian bridge,** and go back to START.

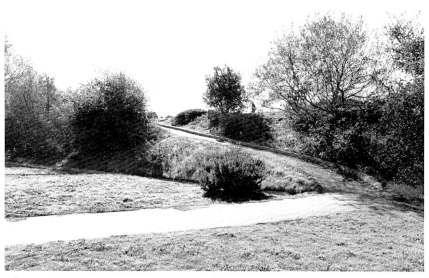

After passing through the Kennan Street gate, follow the asphalt path up to the Riverwalk.

References:

Santa Cruz Sentinel, September 11, 1958, "Branciforte Dresses for Winter."

Santa Cruz Public Libraries, Local History Collection, "History of the County's Emeline Street Complex."

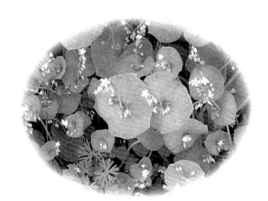

Miner's Lettuce

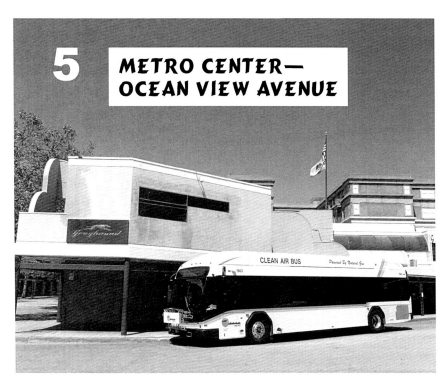

**METRO CENTER—
OCEAN VIEW AVENUE**

3.7 miles / 120 feet elevation gain.

WALK SUMMARY

The METRO bus system provides a good way to get to the walks in this book for those who can decrease their car use. Bus schedules are available at www.scmtd.com.

This walk begins at the METRO Center, salutes a hidden art treasure not in a museum, and takes in one of the grandest views of the river and bay.

GOOD TO KNOW: There are restrooms in the Metro Center, San Lorenzo Park, County Government Center, and in Ocean View Park.

START: The Santa Cruz METRO and Greyhound terminal in downtown Santa Cruz at 920 Pacific Avenue between Pacific Avenue and Front Street across from Elm Street.

◆ **From Pacific Avenue walk east toward the river through the**

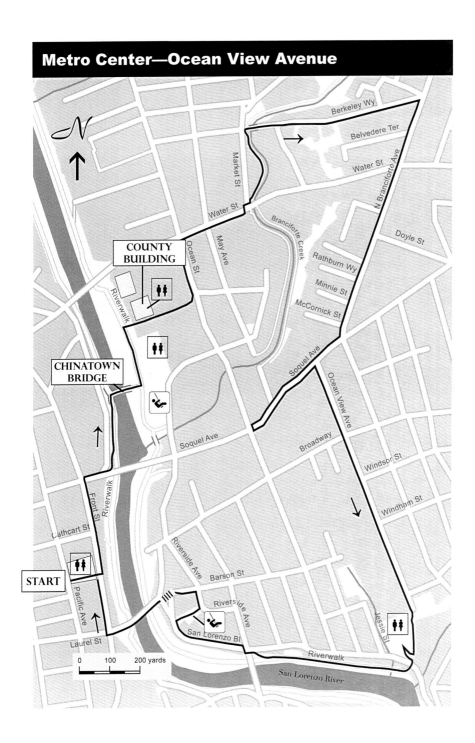

METRO Center station to Front Street.

◆   **Cross Front Street** at the traffic signal.

◆   **Turn left on Front Street.**

◆   **Walk on Front to Soquel Avenue. Cross Soquel, turn right and go to the Riverwalk.**

◆   **Turn left on the Riverwalk before the bridge** and walk north.

◆   **Continue on the Riverwalk under the Soquel Avenue Bridge.**
Check the bridge for the mud nests of Cliff Swallows during springtime. Alongside the path you might notice Sticky Monkeyflower, Wild Roses, or other native plants among the mostly non-native grasses and vegetation.

Local plants and wildlife are highlighted in the progression of mosaics decorating the bridges and walls along the path to your left.

◆   **As you approach the Chinatown bridge over the San Lorenzo River, take the left fork and turn right onto the bridge.**

◆   **Turn left after crossing the bridge.** You are now in San Lorenzo Park. The path continues above the benchlands of the San Lorenzo River.

Ahead is the Santa Cruz County Building. This massive concrete structure is in the aptly-named Brutalist style (I kid you not).

◆   **Turn right at the County Building parking lot and walk through the lot to Ocean Street.**

◆   **Turn left on Ocean Street.**

◆   **Cross Ocean Street at Water Street.** If you enjoy mosaics, check out the one over the bank entrance on Ocean. The real treasure, however, is inside the bank. There are large wall murals signed "S. Hertel," likely by Susan Bright Lautmann Hertel (1930-1993), an artist of some note. Additionally, there is a large stained glass window over the entrance doors from the parking lot. The window is best viewed from the inside from the

Ocean Street entrance so that light is passing through the colored glass.

◆ **Continue east on Water Street.**

◆ **Turn left and cross Water Street at the traffic signal at Market Street.**

◆ **Once across the street, turn right and cross Market Street.**

◆ **Enter the asphalt Branciforte Creek path on the corner.**

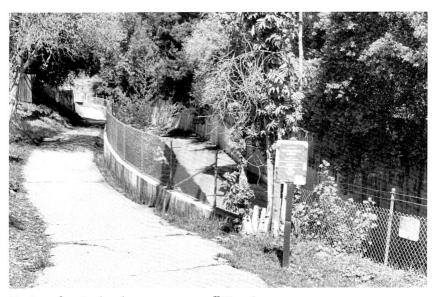

The Branciforte Creek path near its entrance off Water Street.

[See photo above.] As you walk along the path, notice the Miner's Lettuce, a native plant that likes moist areas and provided much needed nutrition to Gold Rush fortune seekers.

◆ **The path returns to Market Street at a pedestrian/bicycle bridge across Branciforte Creek.**

◆ **Turn right and cross the pedestrian bridge.** You are now on Berkeley Way.

◆ **Walk up the Berkeley Way hill.** At the top of the rise be sure to turn around and look behind at the hills of Pogonip and the University of California Santa Cruz.

◆ **Turn right on North Branciforte Avenue.** Look for the 1956 Army Corps of Engineers survey mark embedded in the sidewalk. I have no idea why this marker is here. I suspect it has something to do with the channelization of the San Lorenzo River after the 1955 flood. If you find out, please let me know.

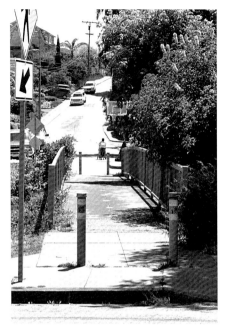

The pedestrian bridge over Branciforte Creek takes you to the hill going up Berkeley Way.

Linger for a minute on the corner of North Branciforte Avenue and Water Street. Across North Branciforte Avenue is a used car dealership in a small tiled-roof building which once served as a gas station. Its stucco siding, square columns and tiled roof are design elements of a typical Spanish Eclectic/Mission style gas station of the 1920s-1930s. The antique gas pumps are long gone.

◆ **Cross Water Street.** Across North Branciforte is the former Branciforte Grammar School, now home to several small alternative schools. It was designed by William Weeks and opened in 1915. In 1917 it represented the Supreme Court in *Mothers of Men*, a silent film about women's suffrage

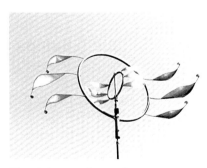

There is beauty all around us.

which was believed lost but subsequently found and restored. The movie, shot mostly in Santa Cruz, features many local places and used Santa Cruz residents as extras.

The area where you are now walking was once the Villa de Branciforte founded in 1797. It was a secular village on the hill facing the Catholic Mission Santa Cruz on the other side of the San Lorenzo River. The settlement had a reputation for tough characters who held bear and bull fights down in what is now San Lorenzo Park. By 1850 the Americans had occupied California, and it had become a state. In 1905 Villa de Branciforte was annexed by the City of Santa Cruz.

◆ **Continue on North Branciforte to Soquel Avenue.**

◆ **Turn right and walk a short distance to a Spanish/Italian**

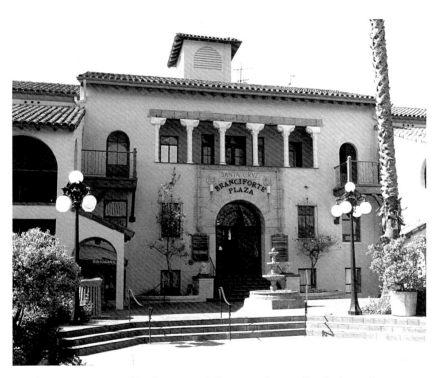

The former Sisters Hospital has been successfully converted to an office facility and restaurant.

style building on the right called Branciforte Plaza (555 Soquel Avenue). The building was built as a hospital in 1928-29, subsequently purchased by the Adrian Dominican Sisters in 1951, and served the city until Dominican Hospital replaced it in 1967. It is worth going inside to see the tile work, wall murals, and old birth records by the restaurant entrance.

◆   **Continue down the hill on Soquel Avenue to Ocean Street.**
As you walk down the hill, notice the large Victorian home across the street behind some businesses.

◆   **Cross Soquel Avenue at Ocean Street.**

EARLY RETURN

If you are ready to return to START, continue west on Soquel Avenue towards town and across the river back to downtown.

◆   **Turn left and walk up the hill on the other side of Soquel.**
We are nearing the 1893 Colonial Revival house at 520 Soquel Avenue with a tower that could house Rapunzel. This was the home of Fred Swanton, a larger-than-life man who played multiple important roles in Santa Cruz for more than 50 years.

Swanton tirelessly promoted Santa Cruz as a tourist destination investing in all manner of businesses including hotels, a movie production company, an electric trolley line, and a seaside resort that eventually morphed into the Santa Cruz Beach Boardwalk. On the way he made and lost several fortunes. In his mid 60s he was elected mayor of Santa Cruz three times. He died in 1940 at 78 nearly penniless.

This elegant house was named "Villa Perla" after Swanton's daughter Pearl. For Pearl's wedding the over-the-top Swanton routed the trolley tracks to the front door of the house from the train station to impress and awe his guests. The large Sequoia behind the house and the Redwood tree in front of it are most likely part of the landscaping for the smaller house (also owned by Swanton) that once stood on this property and was moved to Ocean View

Avenue to give the new home a grand view.

◆ **Turn right on Ocean View Avenue.** We take Ocean View Avenue to its end at Ocean View Park, but there's lots to see along the way.

◆ **Continue to the end of Ocean View Avenue.** The house at 540 Ocean View is the one moved by Fred Swanton to make way for Villa Perla.

When you cross Broadway, you might notice that the crosswalks are not marked with paint at the intersection. Crosswalk paint is applied at some

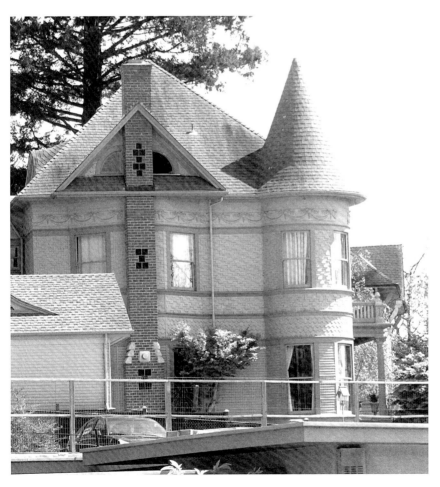

Villa Perla, home of Fred Swanton, tireless promoter and former Santa Cruz mayor.

intersections to alert drivers that people cross the street there. However, every corner is a legal crosswalk even if there is no paint on the pavement. The crossings at such intersections are called "unmarked crosswalks" to distinguish them from "marked crosswalks" which have paint.

Train lovers are in for a special treat at 419 Ocean View Avenue. Both the front yard and the back yard of this home are filled with a creative model train layout (and on special occasions model trains and visitor access). Created by Trevor Park and Eric Child, the miniature Fern Creek & Western Garden Railroad chugs past bonsai trees, over bridges and by settlements to serve logging camps and mines in the early 1900s. Much more fun than grass in the front yard. To learn more visit www.fcwgrr.com.

You will soon pass many posh mansions from the mid to late 1800s. This street with its sweeping views of the ocean and river was the fashionable place to live—the Nob Hill of Santa Cruz. If you want to learn more about these historic properties see *The Sidewalk Companion to Santa Cruz Architecture.*

Note the large multi-trunked tree on the right side of the front yard of 235 Ocean View Avenue. This uncommon tree for Santa Cruz is a Green Ash cited by the City as a Significant Heritage Tree in 1997. Green Ash trees are native to the Eastern United States and Canada. They are not usually planted now because they are susceptible to the Emerald Ash Borer.

◆ **Enter Ocean View Park and walk on the dirt path straight ahead to the top of the bluff** for a lovely view of the Monterey Bay and the San Lorenzo River. Just beyond the obelisk there is a path leading down the hill to East Cliff Drive. [See photo on next page.]

◆ **Take the path to East Cliff Drive.**

◆ **Cross East Cliff Drive at the safety beacon.** This crossing utilizes what traffic engineers call an RRFB (Rectangular Rapid Flash Beacon) to alert drivers. These beacons greatly increase pedestrian safety reducing pedestrian crashes 47% and increasing driver yielding by up to 80%.

◆ **Ascend the asphalt path to the Riverwalk.** Something exciting is always happening on the river. Once we saw a Surf Scoter at this very spot.

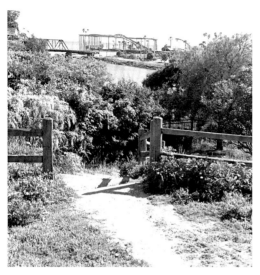

This path starts near the obelisk in OceanView Park and descends to East Cliff Drive.

Another time hundreds of gulls were congregating in the water, then suddenly they took to the air amid a cacophony of calls, circling a bit, then plunged downward to gather again. They repeated this behavior over and over. What will you discover?

◆　**Turn right on the Riverwalk.**

◆　**Walk along the levee path to the exit at the next bridge.**

◆　**Exit the levee at Riverside Avenue.**

◆　**Cross Riverside Avenue.** If so inclined you might take a few minutes to watch skateboarders practice their skills at the Mike Fox Skate Park before returning to the corner to cross San Lorenzo Boulevard.

◆　**Cross San Lorenzo Boulevard at the traffic signal.**

◆　**Turn left on San Lorenzo Boulevard and walk to the entrance of the Riverside Gardens Park** where there are benches and picnic tables as well as a playground.

◆　**Turn right, enter the park, and walk through the park to unsigned Riverside Avenue.**

◆　**Turn left and walk to Barson Street.**

◆　**Turn left on Barson and walk to the end of Barson where there is a staircase.**

◆ **Climb the stairs to a signaled intersection.**

◆ **Cross San Lorenzo Boulevard to the Laurel Street Bridge.**

◆ **Cross the Laurel Street Bridge into downtown.** To your left at the end of the bridge is a complicated assemblage of pipes and pumps surrounded by razor wire. This collection of steel and machinery is what enables the Santa Cruz City Manager to sleep at night. It is the primary storm water pump station that keeps the downtown from flooding.

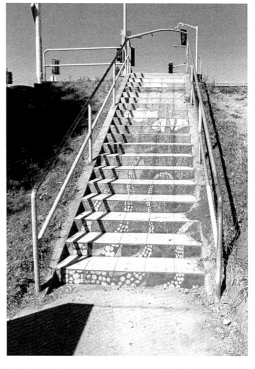

The Barson Street stairs are beautifully decorated with colorful tile.

◆ **Turn right on Front Street. Cross Front and return to** START.

References:

Jones, W. Dwayne, *A Field Guide to Gas Stations in Texas*, Texas Department of Transportation, Environmental Affairs Division, Historical Studies Branch, Historical Studies Report No. 2003-03, 2003.

Chase, John Leighton and Gregory, Daniel P., *The Sidewalk Companion to Santa Cruz Architecture*, Third edition, Edited by Judith Steen, The Museum of Art & History, 2005.

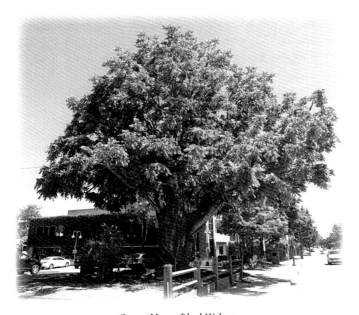

Ocean House BlackWalnut

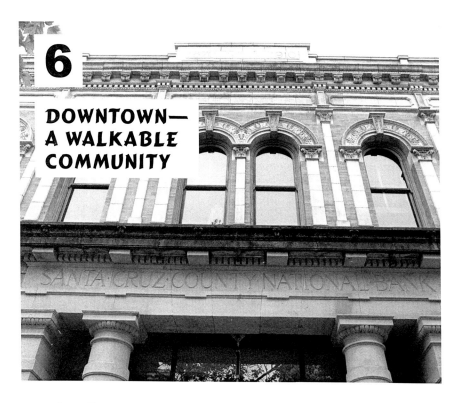

6

DOWNTOWN— A WALKABLE COMMUNITY

1.5 miles / flat

WALK SUMMARY

This walk is a loop along Pacific Avenue and other streets in the downtown pointing out features of interest that are not described in other walks in the book.

Downtown Santa Cruz is a wonderful place to relax at an outdoor café, people watch, check out historic sites, and of course shop. You don't need a guide to walk up and down Pacific Avenue enjoying the ambiance and famously good weather.

Throughout its history, downtown Santa Cruz suffered from alternating fires, earthquakes, and floods which destroyed many buildings in the town center. The present configuration was constructed after much of the downtown was destroyed in the 1989 Loma Prieta earthquake.

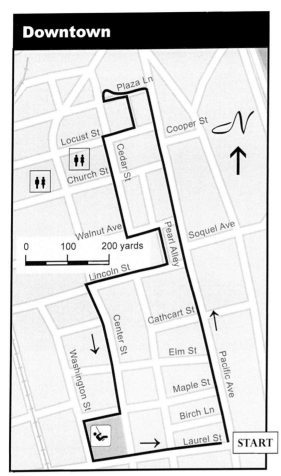

Downtown

Plaza Ln
Cooper St
Locust St
Cedar St
Church St
Walnut Ave
Pearl Alley
Soquel Ave
Lincoln St
Center St
Cathcart St
Washington St
Elm St
Pacific Ave
Maple St
Birch Ln
Laurel St

0   100   200 yards

START

Residents met repeatedly after the 1989 earthquake to listen to expert urban planners in order to determine how to rebuild the downtown. The result was our walkable community design with mixed use residential and retail buildings and wide sidewalks with street furniture and pedestrian amenities.

GOOD TO KNOW: Restrooms at City Hall and the Public Library both a short way off the walk route.

START: Corner of Pacific Avenue and Laurel Street.

◆ **Look around you. Standing on the northwest corner of Laurel Street and Pacific Avenue, we look south across Laurel to two interesting sights.** Directly across the street, high on a building that currently houses a fast food restaurant, is an artfully designed sign announcing "Cimarelli's Corner, Since 1925." The sign commemorates a long-ago moved plumbing service.

Diagonally across Laurel Street and occupying the entire block between Pacific Avenue and Front Street is a curvy building currently housing a restaurant and retail

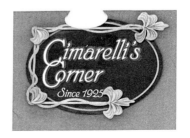

business. The curved showroom windows on each end of the building look like they would be perfect for displaying something large and expensive.

You guessed it. This building, built in 1947, was Bill O'Rielly's Dodge Plymouth Showroom. Can't you just picture a sporty station wagon with polished wood side panels proudly displayed in the expansive window?

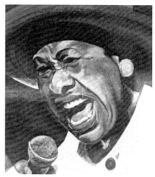

Portion of Jazz Alley mural.

◆ **Walk north on Pacific Avenue**

passing sculptures and several tree-named side streets. On the corner of Birch Lane and Pacific Avenue is the mural "Jazz Alley" by Marvin Plummer, commissioned in 2010 as part of the 35th anniversary of the Kuumbwa Jazz Center just down Birch Lane.

After passing Cathcart Street we see two Art Deco buildings across Pacific: The Del Mar Theater built in 1936 and the former Bank of Italy, now a grocery store. The neon-decorated marquee (best seen after dark) and the tall Del Mar sign command attention. Inside, the mezzanine with its original ceiling lights is alone worth the price of admission. The interior bas-reliefs on each side of the main auditorium screen display Egyptian-looking women

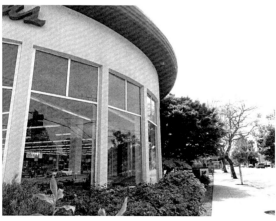

The former auto showroom for Bill O'Rielly's Dodge Plymouth.

with long arms that would make an orangutan jealous. The Del Mar closed in 1999 but reopened in 2001 after purchase by the City and subsequent restoration.

The 1929 Bank of Italy, now converted to an organic foods grocery store, was saved from the wrecking ball in

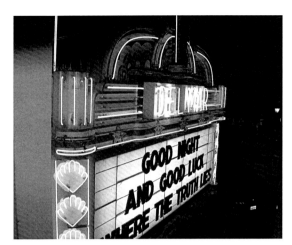

1977 and features lovely exterior decoration including several bas-relief panels.

◆ **Continue walking north on Pacific.** Take time to glance up to see the conquistadores near the top of the Hotel Palomar across the street between Walnut Avenue and Church

Neon fans should be sure to see the Del Mar marquee at night.

Street. We saw them from a distance on Walk 1; now we have a closer view.

Banks played an important role in the life of early Santa Cruz. To evoke trust in potential customers who were used to hiding their money under the mattress or in a coffee can in the kitchen cupboard, architects designed banks

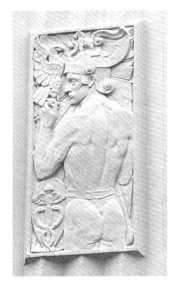

with imposing columns and stonework. In addition to the Bank of Italy where a Greek God moons us from on high, two more historic banks are before us.

At the corner of Locust Street and Pacific Avenue is a massive building built in 1910 as the Peoples Bank. Four huge Corinthian columns face the sidewalk. A bit too fancy to house a sock and shoe shop? Hey, for pedestrians, sturdy shoes and comfortable socks are pure gold.

All that is left of the historic Santa Cruz County Bank across the street at the corner of Pacific Avenue and Cooper Street is its impressive façade. This sandstone structure

Is this Hermes on the front of the former Bank of Italy?

70

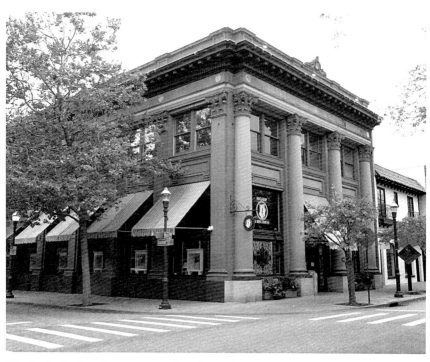

The Peoples Bank with its impressive Corinthian columns.

was destroyed in the 1989 earthquake and the façade preserved. A plaque on the building details its history. Other plaques on the replacement of the St. George Hotel next door at 1528 Pacific Avenue describe the original St. George Hotel, a much beloved Santa Cruz landmark.

Notice the green contra-flow bike lane on the pavement. This street treatment enables bicyclists to legally ride in both directions on a one-way street, making bike travel easier and more efficient.

◆ **Turn left on Plaza Lane** at a break between buildings after 1537 Pacific Avenue. [See photo next page.] You will pass a 1998 mural *Adventures in Paradise* by James Aschbacher depicting Santa Cruz in his whimsical style.

◆ **Walk straight ahead through this hidden plaza to Cedar Street** and check out the mammoth Black Walnut tree fenced off in a parking lot. This tree is all that is left of the extensive gardens of the Pacific

Ocean House, a classy hotel which faced Pacific Avenue. When fungus was discovered in the tree in the 1990s, it was almost cut down. Public outcry led to its being spared. It's a bit funky looking when the leaves have dropped during the winter, but still looks impressive when leafed out. The trunk alone must be sequestering lots of carbon. Thank you tree for helping mitigate Climate Change. Thank you activists for saving this tree.

◆ **After circling this relic return to Plaza Lane and turn right (south) at the bench-lined alley which leads to Locust Street.** [See map]. At the end of the alley there is a mural celebrating the Peoples Bank on the back of the bank building itself. Artist Ann Thiermann has painted several murals in Santa Cruz including one of Native American inhabitants inside the Santa Cruz Museum of Natural History. Her work also graces many other communities throughout California.

◆ **Turn right on Locust.**

◆ **Cross Cedar Street in the marked crosswalk.**

◆ **Turn left on Cedar Street and Cross Locust Street.** Continue walking on Cedar to Church Street.

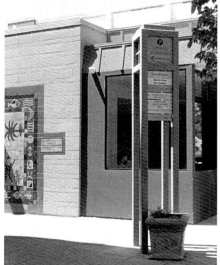

This kiosk marks the entrance to Plaza Lane. Turn left into Plaza Lane here.

◆ **Cross Church Street.** We are now at the Cruzio Building housing an internet provider, the non-profit Ecology Action, and co-working office space. The building used to be the home of the Santa Cruz Sentinel. Before its green building renovation the doors farthest from the corner with large windows above used to be a single giant window reaching all the way to the roof. Inside was the gigantic web press operated at night to print the paper for the next morning. Web presses print on continuous rolls of paper and are often featured in old movies.

Oftentimes walking home from an evening downtown function, I would pause at the expansive window to see the press operating. It was a grand show for this old editor who first saw such a press on a junior high school field trip.

❖ **Cross Walnut Avenue and turn left.**

❖ **Turn right at Pearl Alley** where we see another mural by Ann Thiermann.

❖ **Walk through Pearl Alley to Lincoln Street.**

❖ **Turn right on Lincoln.**

❖ **Cross Cedar Street.** Just beyond the burger place we see the childhood home of actress ZaSu Pitts at 208 Lincoln. Across the street and occupying the full block between Cedar and Center Streets is the Calvary Episcopal Church, the oldest church still standing in Santa Cruz. Its cornerstone was laid in 1864.

❖ **Cross Center Street.**

❖ **Turn left on Center Street.** Occupying the full block bounded by Maple, Center, Washington, and Laurel Streets is the London Nelson Community Center. This former elementary school was

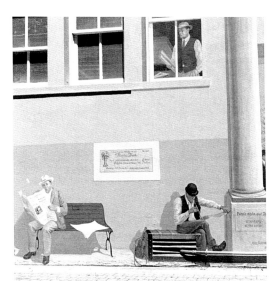

The mural on the back of the Peoples Bank depicts Santa Cruz ca. 1911.

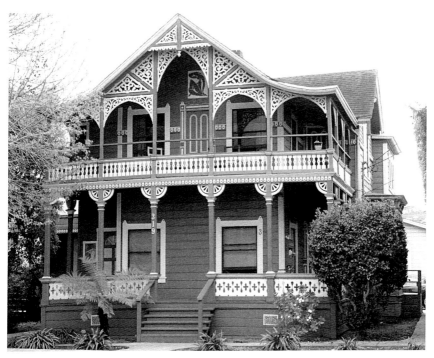

The intricately-cut patterns of the 1887 Four Palms Apartments show scroll saw mastery.

turned into a Community Center which offers classes and hosts community events. It is named after London Nelson, a former enslaved man who donated his worldly goods to the school system after his death in 1860. For more on Nelson and to visit his grave see Walk 3.

◆   **Turn right on Maple Street** to see the charming mural on the back wall of the Community Center facing Washington Street.

◆   **Turn left on Washington Street and walk to Laurel Street.**

◆   **Turn left on Laurel Street and walk back to Center Street.** Notice the intricately cut-out patterns on the 1887 Four Palms Apartments across the street at 319 Laurel.

◆   **Continue east on Laurel Street back to** START.

References:

Chase, John Leighton and Gregory, Daniel P., *The Sidewalk Companion to Santa Cruz Architecture*, Third edition, Edited by Judith Steen, The Museum of Art & History, 2005.

Muth, Deborah, *Santa Cruz Through Time*, America Through Time, 2019.

WHAT IS A WALKABLE COMMUNITY?

A walkable community is one in which it is SAFE and PLEASANT to walk. It is a community where it is easy and safe to walk to stores, the post office, cafes, etc. It is a community that prioritizes PEOPLE over CARS.

WALKABLE COMMUNITIES HAVE:

- town centers
- mixed use development
- public spaces, public restrooms
- complete sidewalk system, benches
- tree-lined streets
- linked streets and trails
- a budget for walkability

BENEFITS OF WALKABLE COMMUNITIES

- increase property values
- decrease auto emissions
- better health
- accessibility for all
- greater safety
- financial savings for walkers

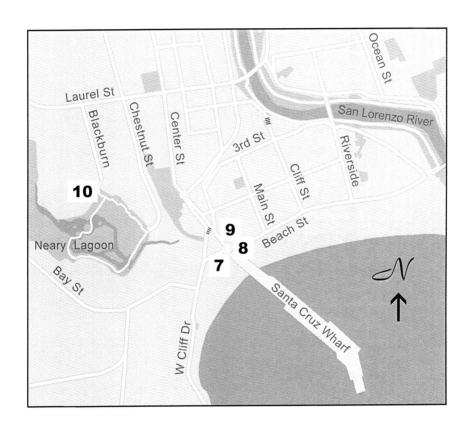

WHARF AREA

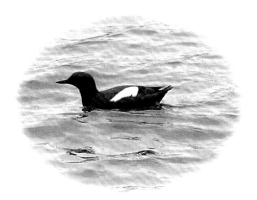

Pigeon Guillemot

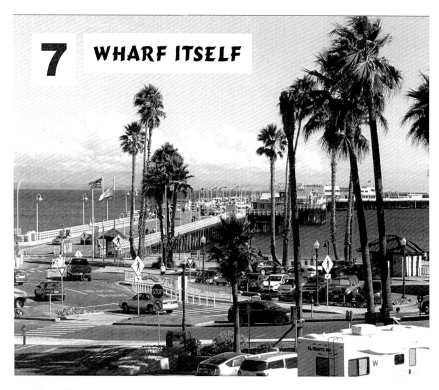

7 WHARF ITSELF

1 mile / flat

WALK SUMMARY

A stroll to the end of the wharf and back offers expansive views of the Monterey Bay and notes the role the Italian fishing community played in the history of Santa Cruz. This saunter gives you the chance to see and hear sea lions up close and personal.

The wharf was built over 100 years ago in 1914 to provide a landing place for deep water steamships. It was the sixth wharf at that general location. A few years after its construction it became the center of the Italian fishing community in Santa Cruz. It was designed to dock steamships and included a warehouse at the end of the pier. Now there are restaurants with incomparable views and kayak rentals.

Brown Pelicans are common on the wharf. They often stand on the railings and watch people fishing in hope of enjoying scraps from fish cleaning. Their

79

The Wharf Itself

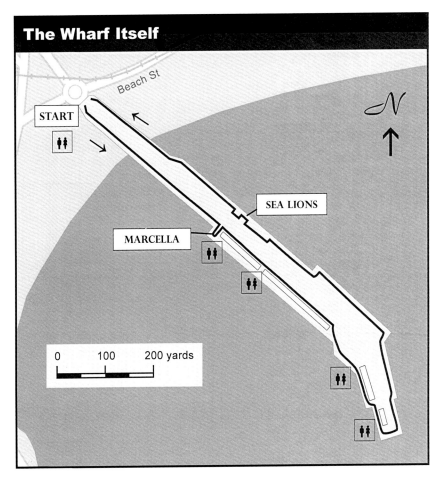

presence is a success story for the Endangered Species Act as Brown Pelicans were on the brink of extinction in the 1970s due to pesticide poisoning. After DDT was banned in the U.S., these birds made a remarkable recovery.

GOOD TO KNOW: Restrooms on Beach Street near start of walk and also on Wharf.

START: Wharf entrance on Beach Street.

◆ **Walk up the right side of the wharf and return on the other side to take full advantage of the varied views.**

80

◆ Sculpture

There are treasures on the Santa Cruz Municipal Wharf among the t-shirt and souvenir shops. Before you enter the wharf, there is a limestone post and lintel construction looking a bit like Stonehenge to your right. The vertical structure is complemented by stone spheres, some in sections like an orange. The sculpture, called "In the Tides of Time," was created by Alan Counihan in 1995. Look closely and you will see both embedded fossils in the rock and a poem in Spanish and English on the inside of the upright pieces.

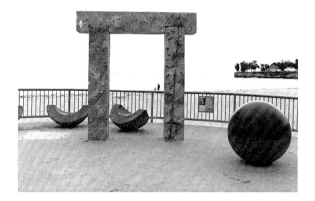

"In the Tides of Time" was created by Alan Counihan in 1995. There is a poem in Spanish and English on the inside of the upright pieces.

◆ Fishing Boat Marcella and Davits

There is a kiosk with information about the fishing history of this area as the Wharf widens about halfway to its end. The historic fishing boat Marcella and a Pelton water-powered davit are displayed. Davits are cranes that lifted the fishing boats in and out of the water. Originally, they lined the other side of the wharf from where the display is located. In a Pelton wheel, energy is extracted from water to perform work, in this case raising and lowering the fishing boats.

When the Santa Cruz small craft harbor was opened in the 1960s, the fishing industry eventually moved there.

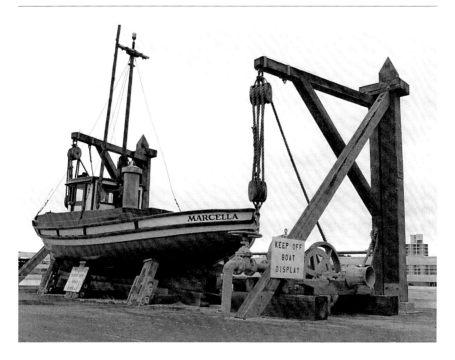

The historic fishing boat Marcella brings us back to the days of the Italian fishing community in Santa Cruz.

◆ Sea Lions

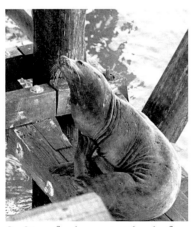

Sea Lions often hang out at the wharf.

That barking sound you might be hearing is coming from underneath the Wharf. Note the railings around five openings in the deck at the end of the wharf where you can observe sea lions catching a few rays or just snoozing. These streamlined creatures love to hang out on the pilings underneath the wharf. In addition to the fenced openings in the deck at the end of the wharf, there is a landing which offers even closer views on our return trip.

Unlike seals which do not have external

82

ears, sea lions have visible ear flaps. They also tend to bark loudly and can walk on their flippers, whereas seals wriggle on their bellies.

From the end of the Wharf on a clear day there are views of Moss Landing (recognizable by the smokestacks of the power plant) and Monterey. Believe it or not you are not looking west to the Pacific Ocean, but south across the Monterey Bay.

◆ **Return to the Wharf entrance on the other side of the Wharf** enjoying postcard views of the Boardwalk amusement park.

◆ **Sea Lions close up**

A short flight of stairs on the leeward side of the Wharf takes you down to a viewing platform where you are just a few feet from basking sea lions. It is a rare chance to closely observe the fur and teeth of these large marine mammals. Note how their flippers resemble the fingers of our own hands.

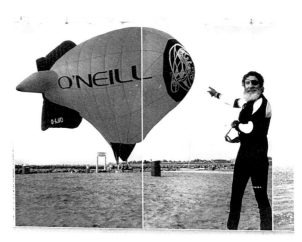

◆ **When you leave the Wharf, turn left and walk up the hill towards the Dream Inn.** On your way stop at the plaque on the wall across the

Jack O'Neill opened a surf shop near the wharf in 1959. Section from a mural by the shop site.

parking lot from the "In the Tides of Time" sculpture to note the spot where Jack O'Neill, inventor of the wetsuit, opened his surf shop in 1959.

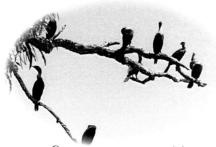

Cormorants above Trestle Bridge

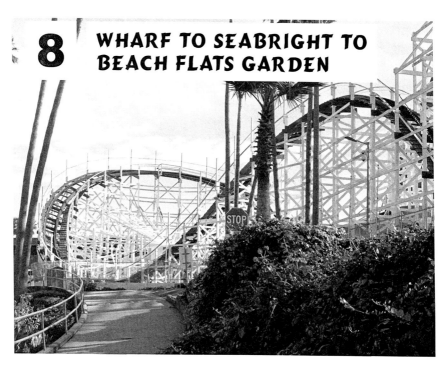

8 WHARF TO SEABRIGHT TO BEACH FLATS GARDEN

3 miles / 120 feet elevation gain

WALK SUMMARY

Go directly to the Boardwalk and collect hundreds of dollars of memories on this historic stroll which crosses the San Lorenzo River, takes a hidden path, and ends at a community garden reclaimed from a trash-laden lot.

GOOD TO KNOW: Restrooms on Beach Street near the start of the walk.

START: Wharf roundabout.

◆ **Walk east on the ocean side of Beach Street from the wharf roundabout toward the Boardwalk amusement park.** On your promenade you will pass Main Beach with its famous beach volleyball courts and bustle of vacationers, if you are walking in the summer or on a fall or spring weekend. If you are lucky, you might even see smiling families chugging to Felton or arriving at the beach in the open train cars of the Santa Cruz Big Trees Railroad. If you do, be sure to wave to the engineer. Souvenir shops and restaurants beckon from across the street.

Be aware of the protected two-way bike lane next to the curb as you walk, and please stay on the sidewalk. Bikes sometimes whiz by at high speed, so take care if you decide to cross the street.

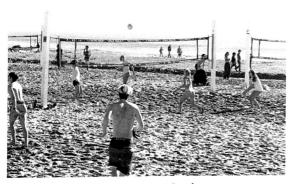

Beach volleyball is popular on Main Beach.

Soon you will pass the Santa Cruz Beach Boardwalk, California's oldest continuously operated seaside amusement park. It was built in 1907 by

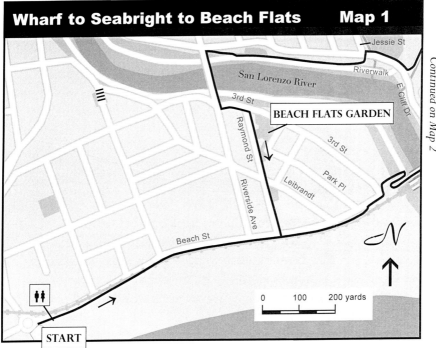

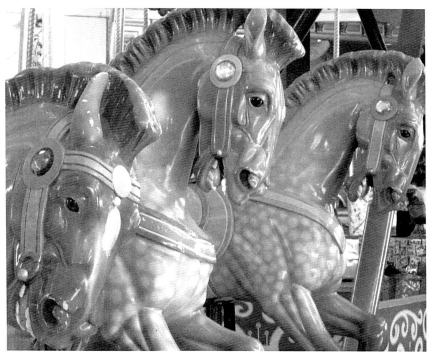

The 1911 Looff Carousel with its hand-carved horses is a treat for young and old alike.

Fred Swanton. Neptune's Kingdom which faces the railroad tracks formerly housed the Natatorium (a heated indoor salt-water swimming pool).

◆   **Stay on the upper roadway alongside the railroad tracks.** The Boardwalk is home to my favorite ride, the 1911 Looff Carousel. Each of the 73 unique horses is hand carved in exquisite detail from multiple pieces of wood and sports a real horsehair tail. Music for the ride is produced by an 1894 Ruth and Sohn band organ and a Wurlitzer 165 band organ. The carousel and the nearby Giant Dipper wooden roller coaster are National Historic Landmarks. The 1924 Giant Dipper, by the way, was built by Looff's son Arthur.

◆   **Descend an asphalt ramp to the sidewalk and follow the signs up to the Pedestrian/Bicycle Bridge over the San Lorenzo River.** You will walk on the edge of the Boardwalk parking lot and switchback up a ramp to the Trestle Bridge.

◆   **Cross the river on the 2019 bike/pedestrian walkway** which is cantilevered off the railroad bridge. It replaced a too-narrow 5-foot wide crossing. The bridge provides a nice vantage point for looking at birds both on the river and in the tall trees on the east bank. (Sometimes frequented by a Peregrine Falcon).

◆   **Follow the ramp up to the street on the east side of the river.** Often Double-crested Cormorants are perched on the trees next to the ramp with their wings outstretched to dry.

◆ **Turn left on East Cliff Drive after reaching the top of the ramp,** and walk a short distance to a painted crosswalk.

◆ **Cross East Cliff Drive.**

◆ **Continue straight on Hiawatha Avenue.**

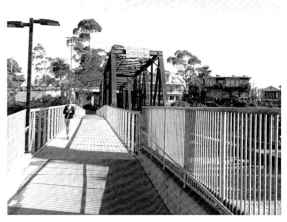

The pedestrian/bike bridge across the San Lorenzo River leads from the Boardwalk to the Seabright neighborhood.

◆ **Follow Hiawatha as it curves first to the right and then to the left passing Cayuga Street and finally ending at a guard rail.**

◆ **Turn left on Mountain View Avenue.** Notice that the name Mountain View Ave is stamped on the curb. The name Anona is stamped on the Hiawatha Avenue side, documenting a name change of the street after the sidewalk was constructed.

◆ **Turn right on Logan Street.**

◆ **Follow Logan to Seabright.** If you look carefully, you will notice you are passing over seasonal Pilkington Creek which flows by the Museum of Natural History before reaching the ocean at Seabright Beach.

◆ **Turn left on Seabright Avenue.** This local commercial area, full of restaurants and shops, was primarily developed in the early 20th century. Seabright was annexed into the City of Santa Cruz in 1905.

◆ **Walk past Hall and Woods Streets to Pine Street.**

◆ **Turn left on Pine Street.**

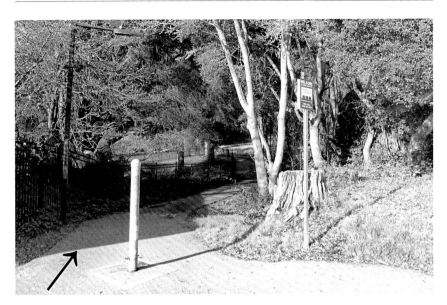

Turn right at this asphalt path leading downhill.

◆ **Turn left facing Cayuga Street and you will notice two other streets at this 5-way intersection.**

◆ **Take the middle street which is Buena Vista** [See map].

◆ **Follow Buena Vista Avenue past Idaho Avenue. Before you reach Logan Street an asphalt path will head downhill on your right.** [see photo].

◆ **Follow the path down the slope.**

◆ **Turn left at the bottom of the slope by a fire hydrant and follow a dirt path along a wrought iron fence.** Active transportation advocates worked hard to keep this path open to the public when nearby property owners wanted to close it. Before the iron fence was installed, a tall board fence created a walled-off space behind which illegal activity could not be seen. The see-through fence and maintenance of the riparian area have increased safety and public use on this important pedestrian and bicycle shortcut.

90

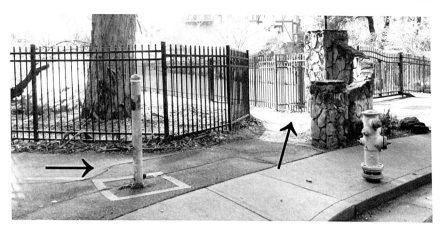

At the bottom of the slope follow the dirt path along a wrought iron fence.

◆ **Turn right on East Cliff Drive at** the marked pedestrian crossing with the flashing beacon.

◆ **Cross East Cliff at the flashing safety beacon** waving politely to drivers so they yield to pedestrians as required by law.

◆ **Continue straight up the ramp to the** Riverwalk. It is always a treat to walk on the levee. Depending on the season and the stars, the bird life varies, but is ever amazing. Across the river we can see the Boardwalk rides.

◆ **Just past an "exit ramp" the path forks. Take the right fork, exit the levee, and turn left to cross the Riverside Avenue Bridge.**

◆ **Cross the Riverside Avenue Bridge.** Here's another chance to check for birds along and in the river and, during springtime, cliff swallow activity on the bridge itself.

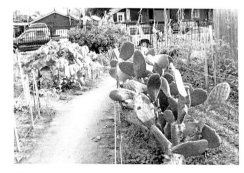

The Beach Flats Garden.

◆ **Cross Third Street at the traffic signal.**

◆ **Turn left on Third Street.**

◆ **Turn right on Raymond Street.** You will soon arrive at the Beach Flats Community Garden and Poets Park. The Beach Flats Community Garden was created in 1994. The murals in the nearby park were created about the same time. The park and garden areas have become the center of this lower-income Latinx neighborhood. The history of the garden and the political struggle to save it in 2016 is the subject of an exhibit in the Santa Cruz Museum of Art and History [see Walk 3]. Panels explaining the mural in the park recount the human and natural history of the Beach Flats neighborhood.

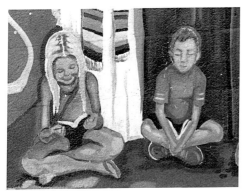

◆ **Continue on Raymond past the Beach Flats Park** with its colorful mural and educational signage.

◆ **Turn right on Beach street and return to** START.

Part of the Beach Flats mural.

Reference:

Department of Planning and Community Development, City of Santa Cruz, Santa Cruz Historic Building Survey, Volume III, March 2013.

9 BEACH HILL

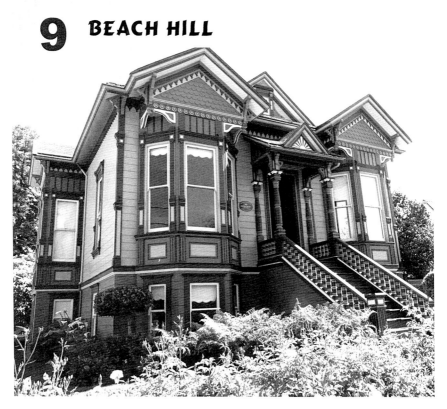

1.5 miles / 80 ft. elevation gain

WALK SUMMARY

I f you are into historic houses, you could get
seriously sidetracked on this walk on Beach
Hill where blue historic plaques and towers
on buildings abound. From Beach Hill you
descend a hidden set of stairs and circle back
to another stairway and a historic bridge.

GOOD TO KNOW: Restrooms on Beach
Street across the street from the start of walk
and at Depot Park.

START: At the northeast corner of Pacific

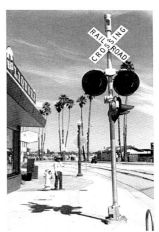

*Start of the Beach Hill walk
across the street from Wharf
entrance.*

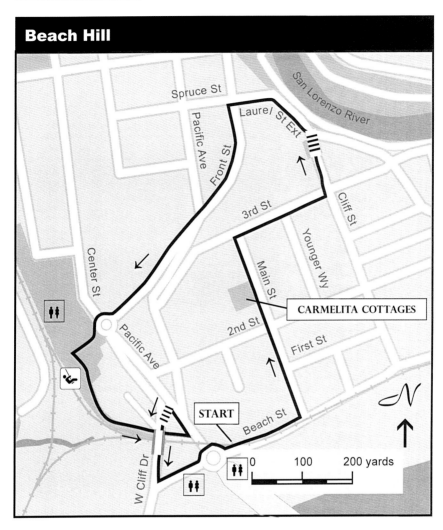

Beach Hill

Spruce St

San Lorenzo River

Laurel St

Pacific Ave

Front St

Laurel St Ext

3rd St

Cliff St

Center St

Younger Wy

Main St

CARMELITA COTTAGES

Pacific Ave

2nd St

First St

START

Beach St

W Cliff Dr

N

0   100   200 yards

Avenue and Beach Street by the fire hydrant. [See map and photo.]

◆ **Walk east on Beach Street to Main Street.** The large hotel with a tower-dome (under construction as this is written) facing Beach Street is the site of *La Bahia* (The Bay), an apartment building constructed in 1926. The tile-adorned tower is the only part of the original building left. The Spanish Colonial Revival building was designed around several inner courtyards with fountains and gardens joined by arched passageways. Although eligible for National Historic Register designation, La Bahia was allowed to deteriorate

94

over the years and torn down in 2020 except for the tower which was incorporated into the new hotel.

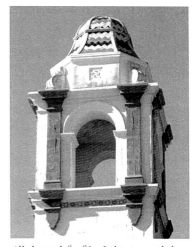

◆ **Turn left on Main Street and ascend Beach Hill.** Once a Native American settlement, Beach Hill now hosts buildings from the 1870s to the present in a variety of architectural styles. Beach Hill was sometimes surrounded by water before the San Lorenzo River levees were built.

◆ **Continue to 315-321 Main Street, the Carmelita Cottages.**

All that is left of La Bahia is its tiled tower.

The Carmelita Cottages consist of six main buildings built between 1872 and 1914. These historic buildings are now operated as a hostel and are located in an approximately half-acre park owned by the City of Santa Cruz. The restored complex with its garden full of heritage trees is a tribute to the perseverance of local preservationists who worked for more than a decade to save the buildings and establish the hostel.

This property was once owned by John-Baptiste Arcan, one of the emigrants stranded in Death Valley on the way to California in 1849. On Walk 3 one can see Arcan's grave and the grave of his daughter Julia, the first person buried in Evergreen Cemetery. Julia, born after the Arcan family reached Santa Cruz, lived only 19 days.

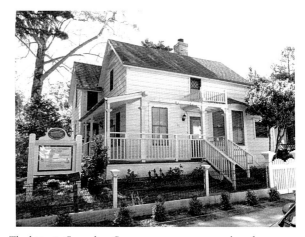

The historic Carmelita Cottages are now run as a hostel.

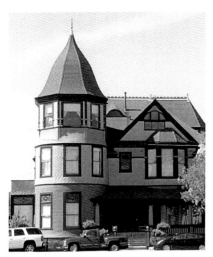

◆ **Continue walking on Main Street to the intersection of Third Street.** Golden Gate Villa, looming straight ahead at 924 Third Street, was built in 1891 for Major Frank McLaughlin, a mining engineer. Designed by San Francisco architect Thomas J. Welsh, who also designed Holy Cross Church on Mission Hill [see Walk 1], the mansion was wired for electricity as well as gas jets for backup lighting during frequent power outages.

Golden Gate Villa stands majestically at the end of Main Street.

Teddy Roosevelt and Thomas Edison were guests in this lavishly decorated home. McLaughlin lived there with his wife Margaret and stepdaughter Agnes who was a toddler when McLaughlin married her mother.

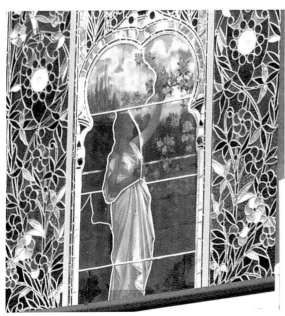

Some say the house is haunted because of the terrible tragedy that occurred there. In 1907, two years after the death of her mother, 33-year-old Agnes was shot and killed by her stepfather while she was taking a nap. McLaughlin then committed suicide by taking potassium cyanide.

Notice the stained glass window on the

This stained glass window immortalizes Agnes.

second floor on the left side of the house as you face it. This window, which is in the stairway to the second floor, immortalizes Agnes. A toga-clad woman, said to be Agnes, is pictured holding a bouquet of violets in one hand and reaching up to pick some apple blossoms with the other. At times when the bushes have been allowed to grow up high, the window is not easily visible from the street.

On the southeast corner of Second and Main Streets there are remnants of a wonderful old neon sign for the long-closed Beach Hill Court, tourist bungalows that are now private residences. The sign was manufactured by the Electrical Products Corporation which was established in 1912 and merged with another company in 1962. I'm guessing this one was made in the 1930s.

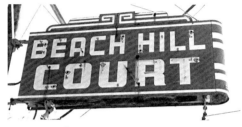

This wonderful old neon sign still survives on Beach Hill.

◆ **Turn right (east) on Third Street and walk to Cliff Street.** Across the street with its entrance at 417 Cliff Street is the Deming House built in 1899 and now an apartment house. Dorothy Deming Wheeler grew up in this house and later built her own home on Spring Street near the Pogonip. Wheeler was the powerhouse who transformed the Pogonip Golf Club into a Polo Club in the 1930s. [See Walk 2.]

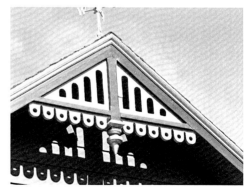

House detail on Beach Hill.

◆ **Turn left on Cliff Street; walk to the end of the street.** Ignore the sign which says "Not a Through Street." It should read "Not a Through Street for cars—Pedestrian Shortcut."

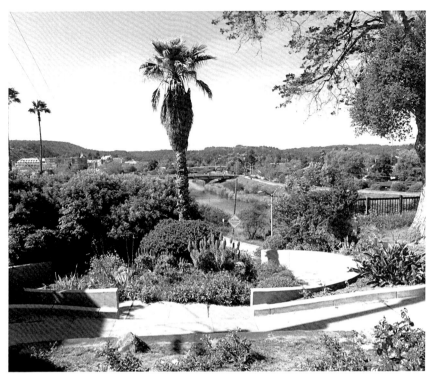

Enjoy the grand view before you descend the Rennie Stairs at the end of Cliff Street.

We can walk down the stairs at the top of the hill [Rennie Stairs].

Pause at the end of the street to admire the huge Monterey Cypress which once stood by the William Rennie mansion built in 1890. This house was torn down in 1970. Also enjoy views of the San Lorenzo River below.

◆ **Descend the curving walk and replaced stairs to Laurel Street Extension which ends at Front Street.**

◆ **Turn left on the sidewalk at the bottom of the stairs and walk to Front Street.** DO NOT CROSS LAUREL STREET EXTENSION TO GO ON THE RIVER LEVEE.

◆ **Cross Front Street** by the sports arena to the murals on the other side of the street.

98

◆   **Turn left after you cross Front Street.** As you walk along Front Street look up to see the rear of the Golden Gate Villa and other buildings.

◆   **Continue straight on Front and cross Pacific Avenue.** TAKE CARE WHEN YOU CROSS PACIFIC AVENUE AS THE TRAFFIC COMING FROM THE LEFT DOES NOT STOP.

As you near the roundabout at the intersection of Center Street, glance up to your left to see the Sunshine Villa assisted living complex on the hill. The original Gothic Victorian building was formerly a private home and then the Hotel McCray. By the late 1950s it had fallen into serious decay and served as the inspiration and model for the infamous Bates Hotel from the Alfred Hitchcock movie *Psycho*. Hitchcock had a home in nearby Scotts Valley and was very familiar with Santa Cruz.

◆   **Walk to the roundabout at the intersection of Pacific, Center, and West Cliff.** It is lovingly decorated with ceramic sea creatures including squid, octopus, and sea stars.

◆   **Circle the intersection on the sidewalk to the entrance of Depot Park.**

◆   **Enter Depot Park.** Ahead is a terracotta-colored building which started life as the freight depot for the Southern Pacific Railroad and was originally located a bit farther north. It now contains restrooms. The passenger depot burned down in 1998.

The giant sculpture of tules ahead on your left celebrates the freshwater marsh plant which played a central role in the local Native American culture. The sculpture, by Carolyn Law, is called "Before Now."

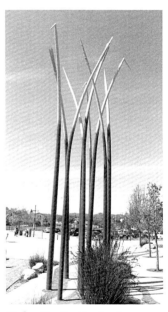

"Before Now" by Carolyn Law celebrates the tules which we see in Neary Lagoon [see Walk 10].

◆ **Take the path to the left between the bike park and the picnic area.** You will walk under the historic Howe Truss Bridge and arrive at the Monterey Bay National Marine Sanctuary Exploration Center (free admission). Note the life-sized sculpture of the whale's tail. This bronze work by Ene and Scott Osteraas-Constable depicts a humpback whale fluke.

◆ **Turn left on Pacific Avenue in front of the Sanctuary Center.**

◆ **Ascend the stairway (Jarboe Stairs) at the corner of Pacific and Viaduct Lane** just past the Sanctuary Center. There is a plaque at the top of the stairs describing the history of the bridge. These stairs were rebuilt in 2000 along with the Howe Truss Bridge. The original stairway led to the c. 1890 second home of San Francisco attorney John R. Jarboe and his wife Mary Halsey Thomas, a writer.

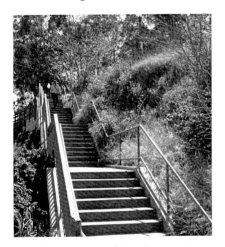

The Jarboe Stairs once led to the second home of San Francisco attorney John R. Jarboe.

◆ **Turn left to cross the Howe Truss Bridge.** The bridge over the railroad tracks is a relatively rare Howe Truss design invented by William Howe, an uncle of Elias Howe, inventor of the sewing machine. This bridge is the last remaining bridge of its type in the state highway system. The original bridge was built in 1918 and rebuilt in 2000 to meet modern earthquake and traffic safety standards. The center span preserves the original wooden bridge supported by hidden steel girders. The rest of the bridge uses new timbers cut to the specifications of the original. Take a minute to admire the view of the Wharf from the bridge.

◆ **Once over the bridge turn left and walk down the hill** to the START at the Wharf taking in a sweeping view of the Main Beach and Boardwalk Casino.

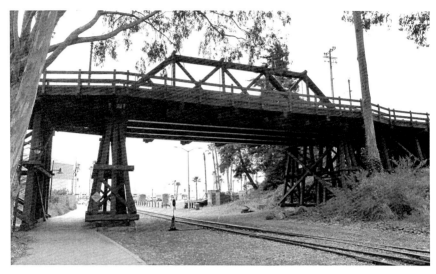

The Howe Truss Bridge is the last remaining bridge of its type in the State Highway system.

References:

Chase, John Leighton and Gregory, Daniel P., *The Sidewalk Companion to Santa Cruz Architecture*, Third edition, Edited by Judith Steen, The Museum of Art & History, 2005.

Dormanen, Susan, "The Golden Gate Villa," santacruzpl.org/history/articles/653/.

Hyman, Rick, "History of the Carmelita Cottages," history.santacruzpl.org.

Johnson, LeRoy and Jean, Julia, *Death Valley's Youngest Victim*, Second edition, 1996.

Martin, Joan Gilbert and McInerney-Meagher, Colleen, *Pogonip, Jewel of Santa Cruz*, 2007.

Wilkinson, Blaize and Weyers, Heather, "The Santa Cruz Super-secret Staircase Tour," (pamphlet) 2001.

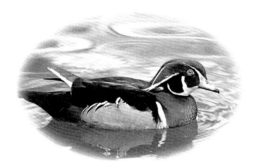

Wood Duck

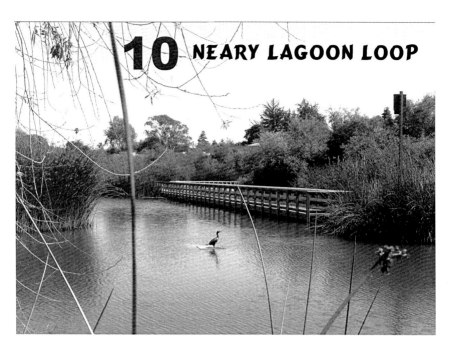

10 NEARY LAGOON LOOP

1.3 miles / mostly level

WALK SUMMARY

The 44-acre Neary Lagoon Wildlife Refuge offers a quiet respite nestled between the noise of the Boardwalk and bustle of downtown Santa Cruz. You are very likely to see colorful Wood Ducks, normally reclusive in the wild, among the more common Mallards and American Coots. Birdwatchers will recognize Pied-billed Grebes, Tree Swallows, and a variety of warblers in the willows.

Budding engineers might enjoy the interpretive panel at the wastewater treatment plant where ducks "swim in the potty water" as my granddaughters used to say.

GOOD TO KNOW: Restroom at the California Street entrance to this city park on Optional Side Trip 1.

START: Entrance to Neary Lagoon at the south end of Blackburn Street. The entrance is on the right, next to where the street is blocked by a gated community. Do not be deterred by unfriendly signage. Blackburn Street

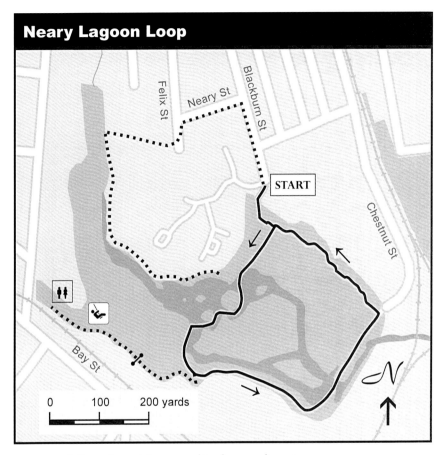

Neary Lagoon Loop

Felix St

Neary St

Blackburn St

Chestnut St

START

Bay St

N

| 0 | 100 | 200 yards |

turns south from Laurel Street and is close to downtown.

◆ **Enter the park and follow the wooden boardwalk to the T intersection** where there is a bench. Listen to the variety of bird songs. You might spot a Black Phoebe, a formally-dressed black and white bird that catches bugs in flight. Neary Lagoon is the remnant of an oxbow of the San Lorenzo River. Twice a year the City hires goats to trim the vegetation here. If you are lucky, you might visit during the foliage feast.

◆ **Turn right. Continue on the boardwalk beneath an arch of native willows.** You soon come to a floating walkway.

The floating boardwalk is surrounded by native tules, a water-loving plant with thick round stems. Native Americans used the tules to construct houses, duck decoys, and even boats. Enjoy the views on either side as you walk across the water.

As you pass a dock that juts out into the water on your right, you might want to walk out for better views. Across the water you can see a wooden dock that you can visit if you take Optional Side Trip 2 described at the end of this walk.

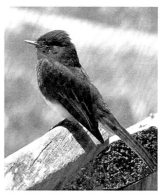

Black Phoebe

◆ **Continue across the floating walkway.** Listen for the metallic call of a Red-winged Blackbird.

◆ **Turn left after you reach dry land** again and continue a few feet to the T intersection with railings coming in on your right.

OPTIONAL SIDE TRIP 1 0.4 mile, 40 feet elevation gain

This short side trip will take you past interpretive displays for the Santa Cruz wastewater treatment plant, a children's playground, and a restroom.

◆ **Turn right and ascend past the wastewater plant towards the tennis courts to a water fountain and a restroom.**

Just before you pass the mural on your left, look to the right for a view of Loma Prieta Peak with its crown of communication towers in the Santa Cruz Mountains. Ahead in raised beds is a native-plant pollinator garden planted by high school students.

◆ **Return the way you came to the T intersection at the bottom of the slope.**

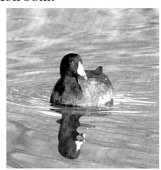

American Coots are dark gray with white bills. They do not have webbed feet like ducks.

◆ **Turn right when you get back to the T intersection.**

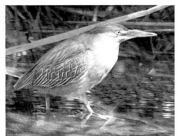

◆ **Continue circling the water on the dirt path.** On poles in the water are nesting boxes for Tree Swallows. These aerial acrobats catch small insects in flight and are fun to watch.

◆ **After you cross over a steel bridge, you reach the Chestnut Street entrance to the park.** Pause on the bridge for good views of wildlife. I have seen Green Herons here.

Green Herons are solitary and secretive.

At the Chestnut Street entrance there is a small amphitheater and interpretive signs. Take a moment to learn more about the historic and natural landscape around you.

◆ **Continue your circle, and turn left to stroll on the zig-zag boardwalk.** About halfway down the path you can see a bat house on a tall

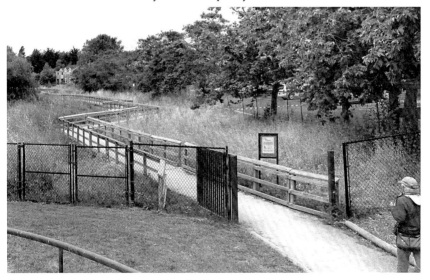

Continue your circle on the zig-zag boardwalk.

pole on your left.

◆ **Continue straight when you come to the T intersection** and go back to START.

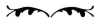

OPTIONAL SIDE TRIP 2 1.1 miles, level

If you would like a further excursion, this mile will give you a chance to spot a Belted Kingfisher from the bank of Laurel Creek on the other side of the lagoon where Laurel Creek tumbles down from Westlake Park. This is the same creek we see on Walk 18. It originates from one of the *Tres Ojos de Agua* noted by the Portola Expedition of 1769.

START: End of Blackburn Street.

◆ **Walk north (straight) on Blackburn Street from the park entrance toward Laurel Street.**

◆ **Turn left on Neary Street and walk one short block until Neary Street ends at Felix Street.**

◆ **Turn left on Felix and walk to the cul-de-sac.** Access to the Sanctuary is through the Cypress Point Apartments parking lot. At the entrance there is a sign designating the Neary's Lagoon Wildlife Sanctuary. The apartments back up to Neary Lagoon, and there is public access along the shoreline of the Lagoon and Laurel Creek.

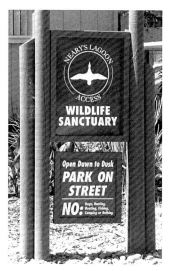

◆ **From the entrance take the right fork in the parking lot and walk past Building 139** and mail boxes heading for the willow tree straight back. Access to the Sanctuary is between units 127 and 129.

From the entrance take the right fork in the parking lot and walk past Building 139 to the access point between units 127 and 129.

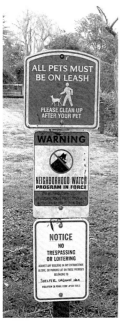

Don't be deterred by unfriendly signs.

◆ **Go past the willow and between units 127 and 129 to the water's edge.** Do not be intimidated by various forbidding signs which tell you there is no trespassing by any building or entrance way. You are not there to hang out by someone's front door. You are there to see the lagoon and its wildlife on property open to the public. **There is public access between the water and the sanctuary marker posts.**

◆ **Turn left when you reach the creek and walk on a grassy path along the water's edge.** Despite the lawn on the apartments side and non-native vegetation in the creek, there is plenty to see and lots of native plants.

Horsetail, a wonderful plant descended from giants in the swamps of the Carboniferous Period 300 million years ago, is found along the banks of Laurel Creek. This plant is high in silica and has been used to scour pots and as sandpaper!

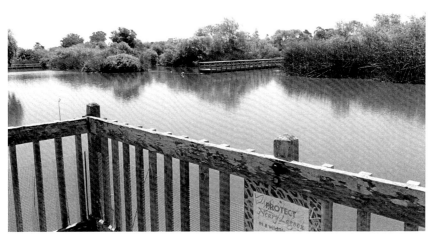

From the Shelter Lagoon side you can see the floating walkway you were just on.

Tules and willows line the banks. The dense tangle of vegetation offers good hiding places for birds and other wildlife.

From this side of the Lagoon you can look back and see the floating walkway you were just on. Listen for the clattering rattle of the Belted Kingfisher. You might even be lucky enough to see one dive for a fish.

Your way continues for about a quarter mile around a bend. Partway to the end a wooden dock juts out into the Lagoon affording you a better view of water-loving birds. I have seen Pied-billed Grebe babies from here.

◆   **When you reach the end, turn around and go back the way you came.**

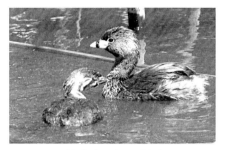

Pied-billed Grebe and baby.

NEARY LAGOON OR NEARY'S LAGOON?

You might see signs calling this park Neary Lagoon or Neary's Lagoon. Which is it? The Neary brothers, James and Martin purchased the lagoon in 1876 and used the property for a dairy and for farming. Early in their ownership it was called Neary's Lagoon. Most frequently it is now referred to as Neary Lagoon.

Reference:

Neary Lagoon Background Information, Final Neary Lagoon Management Plan, Jones and Stokes Associates, Inc. Prepared for City of Santa Cruz Public Works Dept., May 1992.

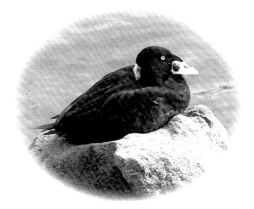

Surf Scoter

RIVERWALK LOOPS

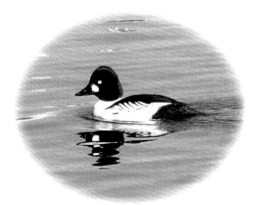

Common Goldeneye

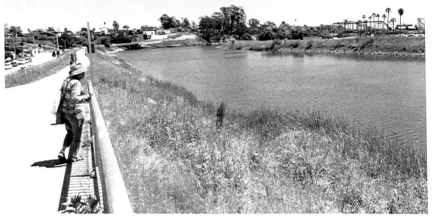

11   BOTH RIVERWALK LOOPS

3.8 miles / flat

WALK SUMMARY

Starting from the west side of the river, we walk north to the pedestrian/bike bridge just south of Highway 1. Then head south on the east bank all the way to the Trestle Bridge near the mouth of the San Lorenzo River. After crossing back to the west bank of the river, we head north back to start. The Riverwalk is popular with joggers and bicyclists including commuters.

GOOD TO KNOW: There are restrooms in San Lorenzo Park and in the Santa Cruz County Government Building midway on the loop. Binoculars are an asset on the Riverwalk.

START: Downtown side of the Chinatown Pedestrian Bridge between downtown and San Lorenzo Park.

◆   **The San Lorenzo Riverwalk Trail can be accessed from any of the bridges that cross the river:** Water Street, Soquel Avenue, Laurel Street, and Riverside Avenue. Additionally there is access from The Tannery Arts Complex, and the three pedestrian bridges. The entire loop is 3.8 miles.

Both Riverwalk Loops

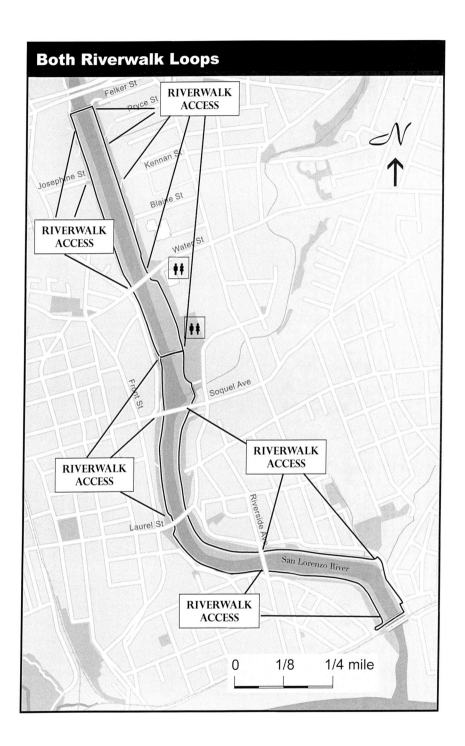

If that distance is not to your liking, you can divide the walk into two loops starting and ending at the Chinatown Pedestrian Bridge between the Water and Soquel bridges. The northern loop is 2.2 miles and the southern loop is 1.6 miles. The Chinatown Pedestrian Bridge is a shortcut between the County Building and the downtown.

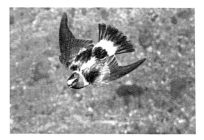

Cliff Swallow

Originally the river channel was much wider and meandered back and forth. Its channel once extended from the site of the post office on Front Street to where the County Building is now. The entire downtown of the City of Santa Cruz is located in the floodplain of the river. The river channel was straightened and the levees completed in 1960 after a disastrous flood in 1955. Some of the bridges were rebuilt in 2004.

Hydrologists divide the lower river into three "reaches." The Estuarine Reach goes from the ocean to the Laurel Street Bridge. The Transition Reach extends from the Laurel Street Bridge to the Water Street Bridge. The Riverine Reach stretches from the Water Street Bridge to Highway 1. The parts closer to the ocean are under the influence of the tides and experience salt and fresh water mixing which influence the plants and animals found in the water and along the banks.

Various unsigned exits along the northern part of the Riverwalk lead to side streets which end at River Street on the west and Ocean Street on the east. Additionally there are exits to downtown full of shops and restaurants.

The San Lorenzo River was named in 1769 by the Portola expedition. The main

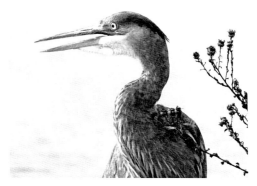

Great Blue Herons can have a wingspan exceeding six feet.

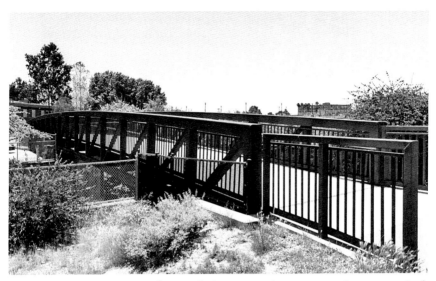

The pedestrian bridge over Branciforte Creek where it joins the San Lorenzo River just south of San Lorenzo Park was the last link constructed to complete the levee path loop.

attraction of the Riverwalk loops is the wildlife one can observe. Perhaps the easiest critters to spot are California Ground Squirrels foraging on the grassy banks. The birds are a special treat. There are water birds in the river, riparian species in the willows lining the channel, and raptors overhead. I have even seen a coyote trotting along the river bank in broad daylight.

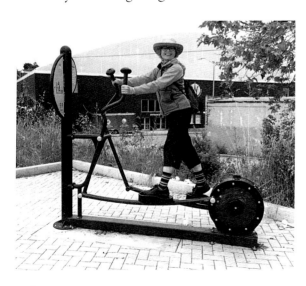

Test your skill on one of the exercise stations.

OPTIONAL EXTENSION: Mosaic bridge stroll   2.2 miles

The mosaics on the Water Street, Soquel Avenue, and Laurel Street bridges creatively depict native plants and animals. These tributes to local talent and our natural resources were shepherded by Mission Hill Middle School art teacher Kathleen Crocetti in 2013 and fabricated by students and volunteers.

You could walk on the sidewalk across one side of the bridge and back on the other side for each of the bridges for an additional workout and art tour. A good way to combine art and fitness.

Colorful mosaics adorn three of the bridges over the San Lorenzo River.

Soquel Avenue Bridge detail.

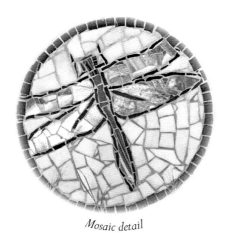

Mosaic detail

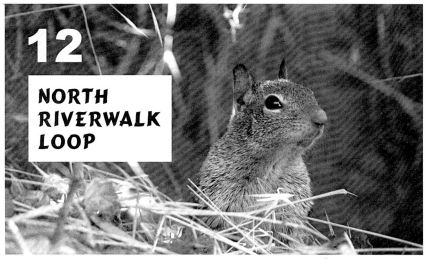

12

NORTH RIVERWALK LOOP

California Ground Squirrel

2.2 miles / flat

WALK SUMMARY

Stay on the west side of the river and walk north to the pedestrian/bike bridge just south of Highway 1. Then head south on the east bank all the way to the Chinatown Bridge back to start.

GOOD TO KNOW: There are restrooms in San Lorenzo Park and in the Santa Cruz County Government Building. Binoculars are an asset on this walk.

START: Downtown side of the Chinatown Pedestrian Bridge between downtown and San Lorenzo Park.

◆ **Head upstream from the start with the river on your right.** From here to the north pedestrian bridge the river channel is braided with less open water than in the southern section. Willows line the banks and often the river itself is difficult to see. In spring and summer invasive (but beautiful) Wild

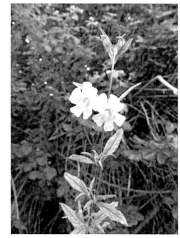

Sticky Monkeyflower

119

North Riverwalk Loop

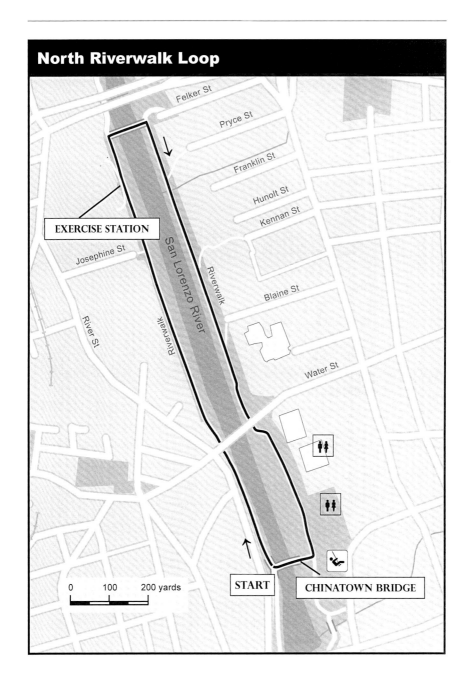

Felker St
Pryce St
Franklin St
Hunolt St
Kennan St

EXERCISE STATION

Josephine St

San Lorenzo River

Riverwalk

River St

Riverwalk

Blaine St

Water St

START

CHINATOWN BRIDGE

0   100   200 yards

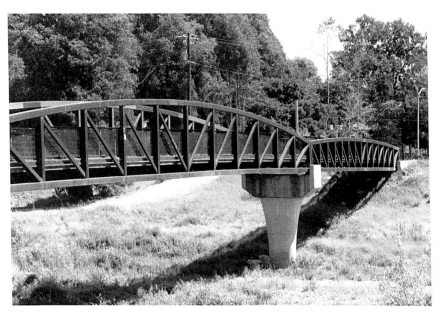

The north pedestrian bridge next to the Highway 1 motor vehicle bridge offers great vantage points from which to view wildlife and riparian plants by the river.

Radish blooms profusely in white and pink.

California Ground Squirrels are found all along the riverbank. These mottled creatures with large brushy tails probably annoy the Army Corps since they burrow into the sandy levee banks. They are fascinating to observe.

To our left on Mission Hill we see Holy Cross Church with its towering steeple. Apartments and trailer homes line the bank. There is an unmarked intersection at Josephine Street

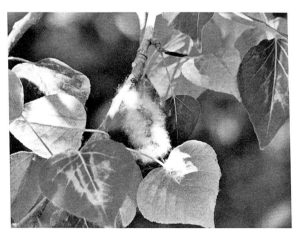

Now we know why they are called Cottonwood trees.

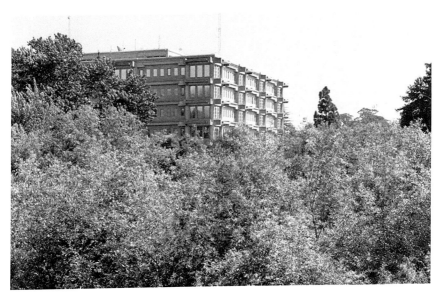

The Santa Cruz County Government Center peeks out from the riparian vegetation as seen from the west side of the river.

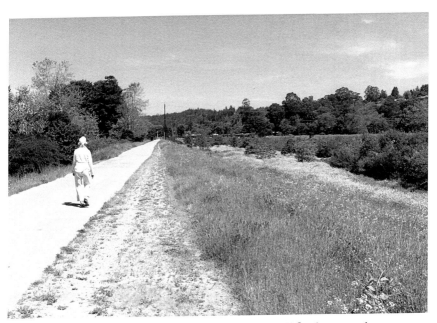

A walk on the levee provides multiple opportunities to view wildlife. It's a great place to get exercise as well.

leading to River Street and, at the north pedestrian bridge, paved paths leading down to a large shopping center. Just before the shopping center is a pop-out plaza with exercise equipment.

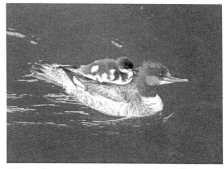

Mama Common Merganzer gives her offspring a ride.

Be sure to pause on the bridge to observe the natural life below. Different times of the year reveal different scenarios. There is higher water in winter as storms and floods scour the channel; in spring ducklings and goslings swim by; each time and season present a unique tableau. There is a good stand of cattail plants just upstream from the bridge.

Heading south after you cross the bridge there are Fremont Cottonwood trees and Coast Live Oaks. If you are lucky, in the spring you might catch the sight of the female Cottonwood shedding fluff to spread its seeds.

As you approach San Lorenzo Park, the fortress-like building with no windows on your left is the Santa Cruz County Jail. Follow the trail under Water Street to San Lorenzo Park. Once in the park you can explore this area to see the Bull and Bear Fight plaque [see Walk 4], bird life, or playground if you are with children.

San Lorenzo Park, adjacent to the County Building (restrooms and rotating exhibits by local artists) occupies the only stretch of the river south of the Highway 1 bridge that was left more open after the flood of 1955. Instead of narrow levees, a series of wide benches was built. The flat benchlands bordered by Fremont Cottonwood trees next to the river and Redwoods above are often used for community festivals. There is also a turf lawn bowling green. Watching this uncommon sport is a rare opportunity for most people.

Cross the Chinatown Pedestrian Bridge back to START.

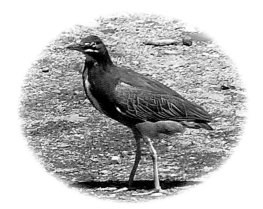

Green Heron

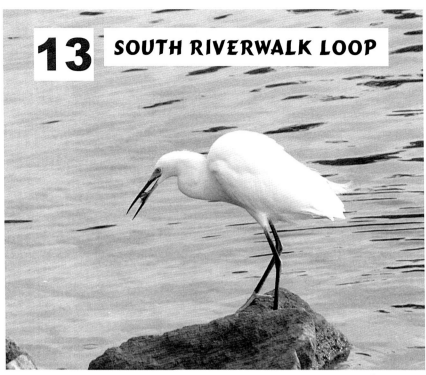

Snowy Egret

13 SOUTH RIVERWALK LOOP

1.6 miles / flat

WALK SUMMARY

We cross the Chinatown Bridge, and walk south to the Trestle Bridge. Return on the west bank back to start.

GOOD TO KNOW: There are restrooms in San Lorenzo Park, in the Santa Cruz County Government Building, and a porta-potty at Front and Laurel Streets. Binoculars are an asset on this walk.

START: Downtown side of the Chinatown Pedestrian Bridge between downtown and San Lorenzo Park.

◆ **Cross the Chinatown Pedestrian Bridge and head downstream on the park side of the river.** Be sure to pause on the bridge to observe the animal life. Often there is a Red-tailed Hawk perched in the tall trees just over the river in the park.

125

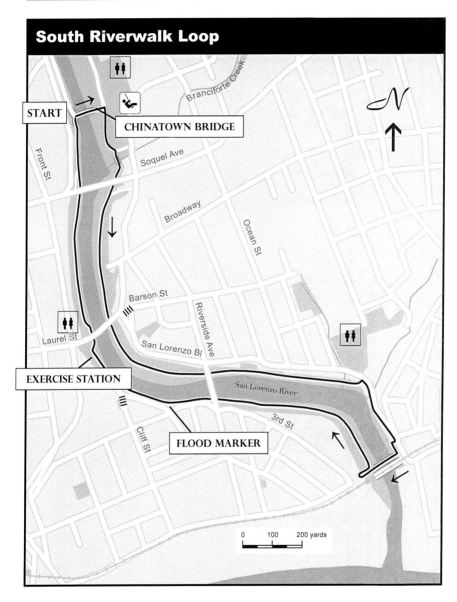

South Riverwalk Loop

START

CHINATOWN BRIDGE

Branciforte Creek

Front St

Soquel Ave

Broadway

Ocean St

Barson St

Riverside Ave

Laurel St

San Lorenzo Bl

EXERCISE STATION

San Lorenzo River

3rd St

Cliff St

FLOOD MARKER

N

0   100   200 yards

After a short distance you cross another pedestrian/bike bridge over Branciforte Creek. At its juncture with the river, Branciforte Creek is encased in concrete walls. We investigate its more natural upstream bed on Walk 4. The Branciforte Creek Bridge was the last link installed in the continuous Riverwalk Loop Trail. Before it was completed in 2017, people had to leave the levee path, cross busy Soquel Avenue, and then return to the levee.

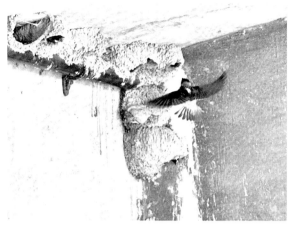

Nearing the Laurel Street and Riverside Avenue Bridges are our best chances to see Cliff Swallows. From about mid-

Cliff Swallows are fascinating to watch as they scoop up mud, build their nests, and raise their babies.

March through summer these birds build nests attached to the bridges. If you are there during nest building, you can see the parents scoop up mud from the river bank as they build. Later on you can spot baby birds peeking out from mud nests. The swallows catch insects in mid flight as they dart around like miniature fighter jets.

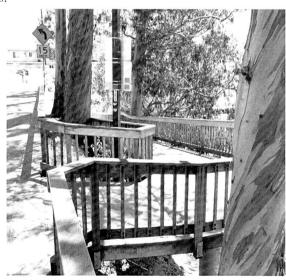

Once south of the Laurel Street Bridge there are fewer trees and a much wider channel. Below the Riverside Avenue Bridge gulls often congregate. The banks are more open. Bird life takes a definite tidal turn.

On the bank just before the Riverside Avenue Bridge it's always fun to watch

The entrance to the ramp leading from East Cliff Drive to the pedestrian/bicycle bridge near the river mouth.

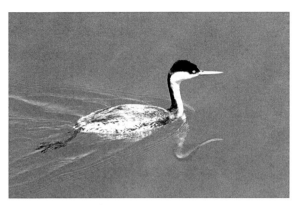

Western Grebes dive for fish and amphibians.

the skateboarders at the Mike Fox Skate Park.

Ahead we can see the Giant Dipper at the Boardwalk and the Trestle Bridge near the river mouth. The view from the bridge is awesome. Below, one often can see sea lions, seals, Common Goldeneyes, and sometimes above, a peregrine falcon.

We trudge up the hill to the Trestle Bridge and find the ramp with its wooden railing between tall Eucalyptus trees. [see photo p. 127]. Don't forget to glance up. Double-crested Cormorants often perch in these trees.

From the bridge there are spectacular views to the river mouth and also upstream. Eventually this bridge will be part of the Rail Trail and Monterey Bay Scenic Sanctuary Trail skirting the entire Monterey Bay.

Once on the west bank of the river head north again.

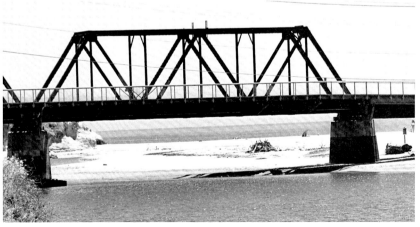

When you cross the pedestrian bridge cantilevered off the Trestle Bridge, look for Double-crested Cormorants perched in the Eucalyptus trees on the east bank.

Near the junction of Third and Leibrandt Streets is a small plaza with a marker showing the height of the 1955 flood. Wow, that was a lot of water! Soon you will pass the Rennie Stairs from Cliff Street which we descend on Walk 9.

Shortly you will pass under the Riverside Avenue Bridge again. Notice the tethered logs along the bank. They are secured there to provide hiding places for young fish. The San Lorenzo River used to attract crowds of people to fish for Coho Salmon and Steelhead. No more. Keeping big logs in the riverbed is a small step toward restoration of the habitat which supports a healthy fish population.

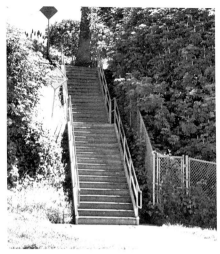

We pass the Rennie Stairs that we descended on Walk 9 coming down from Cliff Street.

Near here you might also see some Buffleheads in winter. These small diving ducks are some of the cutest birds ever. The striking black and white breeding plumage and white back of the head of the males make them easy to identify. They can often be seen in winter and spring on the west side of the river just upstream from the Riverside Avenue Bridge. Don't you just love their name!

South of the Laurel Street Bridge is another exercise plaza. The willows become more dense as you head toward the Soquel Avenue Bridge. Soon you will be back to START.

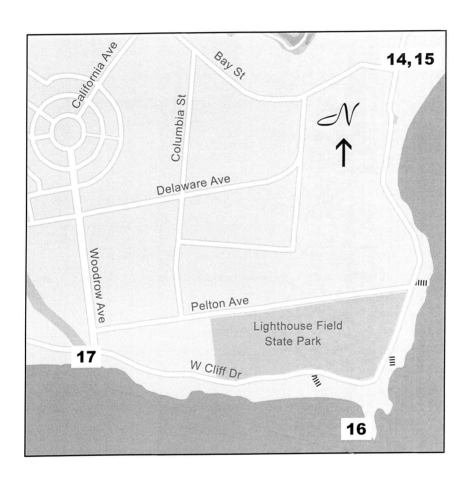

California Ave

Bay St

Columbia St

14,15

N

Delaware Ave

Woodrow Ave

Pelton Ave

Lighthouse Field
State Park

17

W Cliff Dr

16

WEST CLIFF AND THEREABOUTS

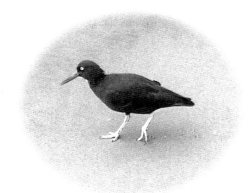

Black Oystercatcher

14 WEST CLIFF TO THE END AND BACK

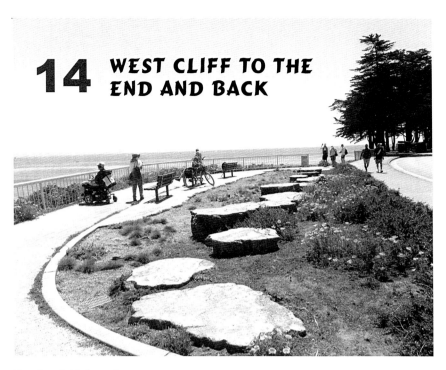

5 miles / 40 feet elevation gain

WALK SUMMARY

The not-to-be-missed stroll along West Cliff Drive in Santa Cruz is a scenic classic. Here are expansive Bay views, sea birds galore, and local color. One may either walk the entire distance from the end of Bay Street to Natural Bridges State Beach (a round trip distance of 5 miles with 40 feet of elevation gain) or break up the walk into smaller segments. We have described four walks along West Cliff Drive in the following pages.

GOOD TO KNOW: Restrooms located across the street from Lighthouse Point and at Natural Bridges State Beach.

START: Bay Street and West Cliff Drive.

Walking along West Cliff can confuse our poor brains which tell us the Pacific Ocean is to the west. But here, along West Cliff Drive the Monterey Bay and Pacific Ocean are to the south! The first time I saw this vista, the coast was clad in fog, and I saw no land as I looked out to sea. The next time I looked

133

out, I saw land! Hills where I expected to see endless ocean stretching all the way to Asia. It's fun to tell visitors that the land they see across the Bay is Hawaii, but of course, it's Monterey. We are looking south.

Spread before you is the Monterey Bay National Marine Sanctuary, designated in 1992 as an underwater national park bigger than Yosemite. It is an amazingly rich biological habitat where one can spot sea lions, dolphins, seals, sea otters, and even migrating whales right from the multiuse path along the bluff tops. To learn more about the wonders of the Sanctuary visit the Monterey Bay Sanctuary Exploration Center across the street from the Municipal Wharf [see Walk 9].

Along West Cliff Drive there are a number of conveniently-placed benches from which to watch the ever-changing pageant of the Monterey Bay with its sailboats, surfers, and seals.

◆   **To enjoy this walk, just follow the path along the shoreline. No navigation needed. There are detailed descriptions of coastal segments in the shorter walks following.**

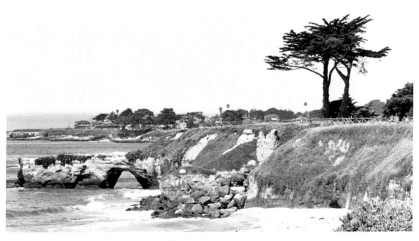

Sea arch by Its Beach along West Cliff Drive.

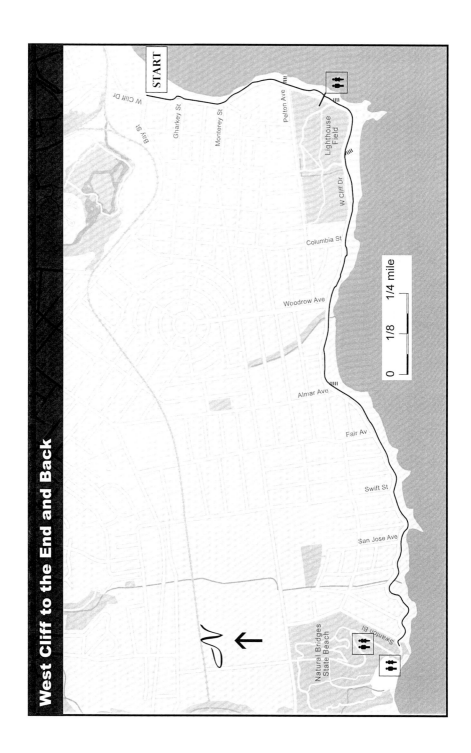

START

W Cliff Dr

Bay St
Gharkey St
Monterey St
Pelton Ave

Lighthouse
Field

W Cliff Dr

Columbia St

Woodrow Ave

0   1/8   1/4 mile

Almar Ave

Fair Av

Swift St

San Jose Ave

Swanton Bl

Natural Bridges
State Beach

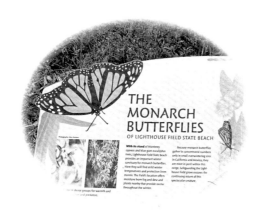

Butterfly Sanctuary

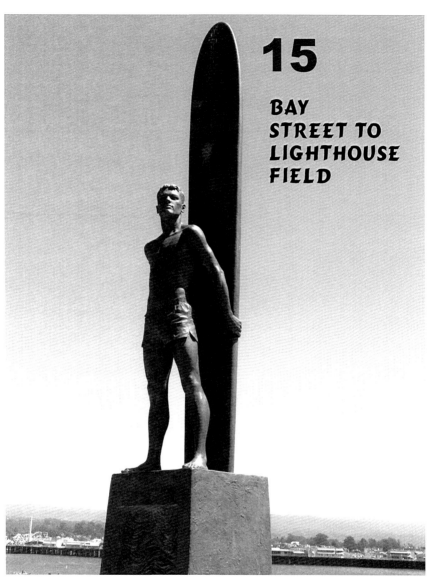

15

BAY STREET TO LIGHTHOUSE FIELD

2.2 miles / 20 feet elevation gain

WALK SUMMARY

We start along the coast with great views of the Monterey Bay and Wharf, cross West Cliff Drive for a quiet stroll through a butterfly sanctuary, then back to start.

Bay Street to Lighthouse Field

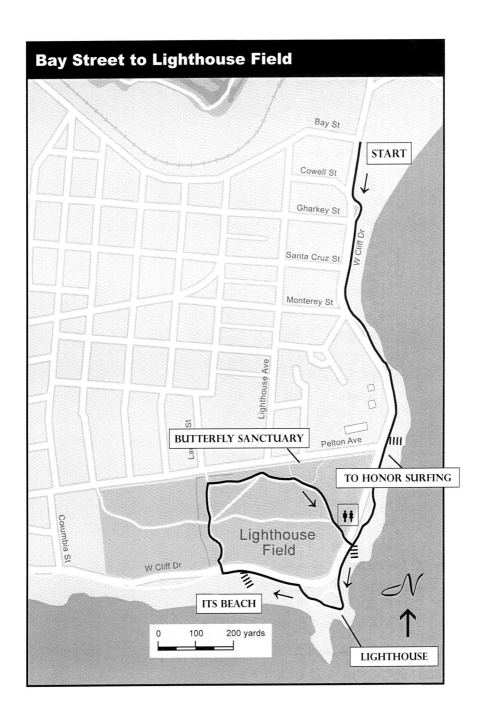

START

Bay St

Cowell St

Gharkey St

Santa Cruz St

Monterey St

W Cliff Dr

Lighthouse Ave

BUTTERFLY SANCTUARY

Pelton Ave

TO HONOR SURFING

Columbia St

Lighthouse Field

W Cliff Dr

ITS BEACH

0   100   200 yards

LIGHTHOUSE

N

GOOD TO KNOW: Restrooms located across the street from Lighthouse Point.

START: Bay Street and West Cliff Drive.

◆　**Walk along the coast away from the Wharf to a pocket park across from the intersection of West Cliff with Cowell Street.** If you take out a compass, you will discover you are walking south. Right from the start one is caught up in the directional confusion that exists in the City of Santa Cruz. Because of the ins and outs of the coastline, you start out walking south to proceed northward up the coast! After you pass Lighthouse Point, the path heads to the west as you continue "north." Confused? Not to worry. You are not in the Twilight Zone; it's just normal Santa Cruz.

This small park has wonderful views of the Wharf and Boardwalk. Take a few minutes to admire the scenery. In addition to the Wharf and Boardwalk, you can see the shops on Beach Street and the Santa Cruz Mountains behind them all. On the skyline behind the Wharf you can see Loma Prieta Peak crowned by communication towers on the summit ridge of the Santa Cruz Mountains. Cowell's Beach, directly below you is popular with beginning surfers and surfing schools.

At the corner of Santa Cruz Street and West Cliff Drive is Epworth-by-the-Sea, built in 1887. This house and others extending to Lighthouse Field are the remnants of a neighborhood once known as "Millionaires Row" or "Millionaires Road" a district of stately summer homes facing the ocean built between 1887 and 1910 by the super wealthy. Most of these lavish homes occupied large properties which stretched from what was called Cliff Drive to Lighthouse Avenue, a full block.

As you near Lighthouse Field, you can see across the road the complex of the Shrine of St. Joseph, Guardian of the Redeemer. That property includes not only the chapel but also the Mediterranean style Davis house built in 1912, and Rutherglen Terrace a Victorian house with a tower, built in 1893 for James and Louise McNeil. James McNeil was president of the Santa Cruz Electric Light and Power Works. Inside the shrine is a delightful coffee shop surrounded by grounds with gardens and a fountain perfect for tranquil relaxation and conversation.

During your walk you will pass three sets of stairs leading down to pocket beaches or rocks providing access for surfers and other ocean users. If the tide is out, more enthusiastic walkers will have several opportunities to explore these staircases. Don't hesitate to run up and down them if you feel energetic.

Stop to admire the bronze statue, "To Honor Surfing" (1992) by Tom Marsh which depicts a 1930s surfer, sans wetsuit with his longboard. Surfing has been a part of Santa Cruz since 1885 when three Hawaiian princes introduced the sport to the community. When you reach the lighthouse, you can see a plaque in their honor outside the building.

Be sure to look for sea otters in the kelp beds. These oh-too-cute endangered mammals are frequently seen from the West Cliff path. Their thick fur coats keep them warm in this cold water, but made sea otters the target of fur hunters in the 19th century when they were almost hunted to extinction. Otters are often seen lying on their backs in the water, sometimes with a rock on their chests, on which they crack hard-shelled seafood.

Just ahead you can see the small brick lighthouse. Before you reach the lighthouse, you pass a memorial to surfers who have died on the waves. Across the street are public restrooms.

Lighthouse Point, which juts out into the bay, hosted its first lighthouse in 1870 when a lard-oil lamp was lit on January 1 of that year. Ten years

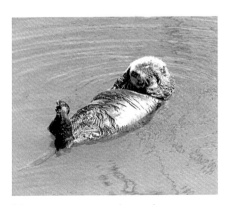

later the lighthouse keeper, Adna Hecox, received orders to replace the clear lamp with one that shone red to distinguish the Santa Cruz light from other nearby lighthouses. When Hecox died in 1883 at the age of 77, his 29-year-old daughter, Laura Hecox, was appointed lighthouse keeper.

The present red brick lighthouse was constructed in 1967 by Chuck

It's a treat to spot an endangered sea otter.

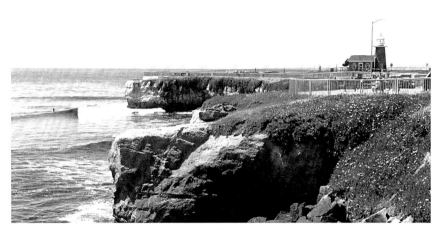

Lighthouse Point juts out into the Bay. The Surfing Museum inside the current lighthouse is full of interesting exhibits.

and Esther Abbott as a memorial to their 18-year-old son Mark who died in a surfing accident. Until this lighthouse was built, there hadn't been a lighthouse there since the 1940s.

◆ **As you enter the park where the lighthouse is located, walk to the railing around the point which looks down on Steamer Lane for the best free show in town except for City Council meetings.** Here expert surfers dance with the ocean carving a sequence of S curves as they speed toward the shore.

The lighthouse itself is now a Surfing Museum. Inside are vintage surfboards, surfboards bitten by sharks, and loads of historic photographs. Many of the docents are long-time surfers who remember the old days. It's your chance to ask questions. Don't overlook the historic plaques outside.

◆ **Continue on West Cliff Drive past Lighthouse Point.** A bronze plaque honoring the service of the African American 54th Coast Artillery Regiment stationed at Lighthouse Field during World War II is located near a bench a short distance past the lighthouse. The plaque is surrounded on three sides by a metal railing.

◆ **Continue on West Cliff paralleling Lighthouse Field across**

the street. If only the landscape could talk. This field, now managed by State Parks, has an interesting history. It has been in turn part of a private estate,

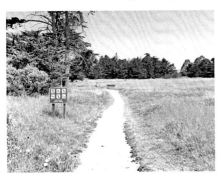

Cross West Cliff and walk into Lighthouse Field on the dirt path.

a camp for an Afro-American artillery regiment during the Second World War (before the military was integrated), and the site of multiple development battles in the 1960s and 1970s that culminated with a political change of direction in Santa Cruz. As you walk through this peaceful field today, give thanks to the many environmentalists who prevented this grassland from becoming acres of parking surrounded by hotels and shops.

◆ **Cross West Cliff Drive on the painted crosswalk** just beyond the lighthouse [see map on p. 138 and photo above on this page]. Those who want more of a workout can jog up and down the stairs to Its Beach.

◆ **Walk into Lighthouse Field on the dirt path leading away from the shoreline.**

◆ **Continue straight at a wide 5-way trail junction with a bench and a very large Cypress tree.** On the way look for raptors near the tops of the tall trees. I have seen Peregrine Falcons, Red-shouldered Hawks and Red-tailed Hawks here. American Kestrels often hover above the grassland.

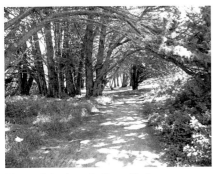

This path leads to the Butterfly Sanctuary.

◆ **Turn right on a smaller path beyond the trail junction, and walk into a Cypress grove.** This cool, quiet place invites contemplation and

142

careful observing. Stay on the path. There is poison oak here.

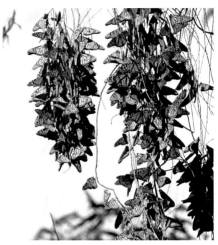

◆ **Keep straight as informal paths come in on either side. Soon you will reach a single-wire enclosure around a Butterfly Sanctuary.** Migrating monarch butterflies overwinter in Santa Cruz and other locations along the Central Coast. Look for them between November and January in the cypress and eucalyptus trees in the fenced off area. Although the

Clusters of over-wintering Monarchs.

numbers of overwintering monarchs has declined drastically in the last few years, this site is still ranked as the 7th most important for restoration out of 111 overwintering sites in California.

◆ **From the butterfly trees walk back to West Cliff Drive on the path which ends at restrooms and a food vendor.**

◆ **Cross the street and turn left on the West Cliff path to** START.

References:

Chase, John Leighton and Gregory, Daniel P., *The Sidewalk Companion to Santa Cruz Architecture*, Third edition, Edited by Judith Steen, The Museum of Art & History, 2005.

Perry, Frank, *Lighthouse Point, Illuminating Santa Cruz*, Otter B. Books, 2002.

Pelton, Emma, et al., "Monarch Butterfly Overwintering Site Management Plan for Lighthouse Field State Beach," October 2017.

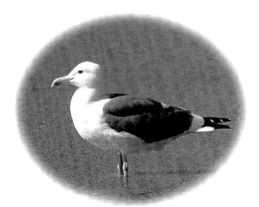

Western Gull

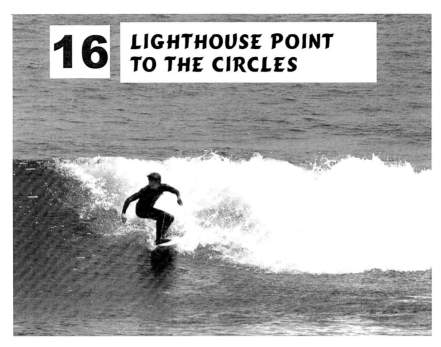

16 LIGHTHOUSE POINT TO THE CIRCLES

2.6 miles / 50 feet elevation gain

WALK SUMMARY

After a short walk on the West Cliff path, we follow a seasonal creek to the interesting Circles neighborhood, returning to West Cliff on a historic streetcar route.

GOOD TO KNOW: Restrooms across from Lighthouse point and at the Garfield Library.

START: Lighthouse Point

◆ **From Lighthouse Point walk up the coast with the ocean on your left to Woodrow Avenue.**

Notice the piles of rocks (riprap) armoring the coast as you proceed. Riprap is placed along the coast to decrease erosion from waves and winter storms. Eventually the ocean will win. Rising sea levels coupled with storms are changing our coastline.

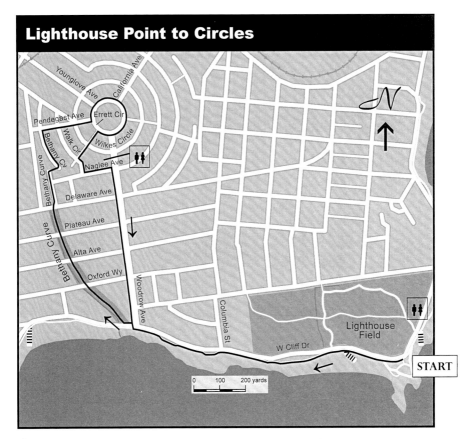

Lighthouse Point to Circles

◆ **Cross West Cliff to the west corner of Woodrow Avenue.**

Why is Woodrow so wide? The Santa Cruz, Garfield Park, and Capitola Electric Railway built in 1891 used to run down this street then named Garfield. During replacement of a water main on Laurel Street in 2005, engineers found these streetcar wheels (see photo next page).

◆ **Take the dirt path leading north through the park area.** This is Bethany Curve, a riparian corridor popular with bird watchers and those out for a neighborhood stroll. The path takes you across four streets: Oxford Way, Alta Avenue, Plateau Avenue, and Delaware Avenue. Beside the path between West Cliff and Delaware are several dog agility structures your pet might enjoy or ignore.

146

◆ After crossing Delaware continue on the street named Bethany Curve all the way to where it ends. You will notice a narrow walkway on your right.

◆ Turn right and in a few steps you will emerge on a street also called Bethany Curve.

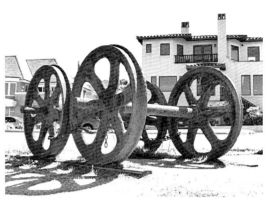

An electric streetcar used to run down the center of Woodrow Avenue.

◆ Turn left and take Bethany Curve to Pendegast Avenue.

◆ Turn right on Pendegast and go past Walk Circle and Wilkes Circle to Errett Circle. You are now in the "Circles" neighborhood, a landmark for amateur pilots flying overhead. This neighborhood of

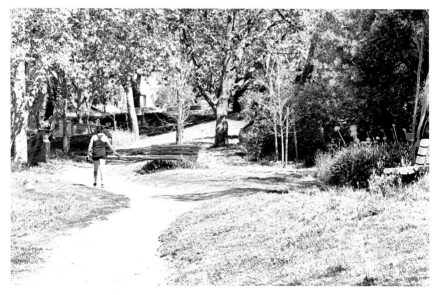

Bethany Curve is a leafy corridor leading from the Circles neighborhood to West Cliff Drive.

concentric circles was built in the 1890s and consisted of canvas tents and small cottages surrounding a church. The first church here had a 100-foot bell tower. It is said that when the bell rang, people gathered up their families and Bibles and walked up the streets and pathways making up the spokes of the wheel to the church in the center.

◆ **Take a quick spin to the left (clockwise) around Errett— the innermost circle—to the alley between 512 and 510 Errett making almost a complete circle.**

◆ **Turn left and walk down the alley crossing Wilkes Circle and ending at Walk Circle.** Imagine you are returning to your tent cabin after a camp meeting at the tabernacle.

◆ **Turn left on Walk Circle to Naglee Avenue.**

◆ **Turn left on Naglee Avenue and walk to Woodrow Avenue.** On the corner of Naglee and Woodrow is the Garfield Park Branch

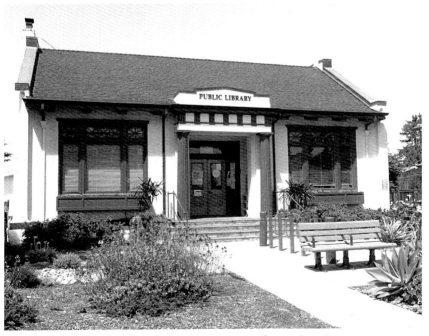

The Garfield Park Library was built in 1915 with a grant from Andrew Carnegie.

Library, designed by William Weeks and built in 1915. Steel magnate and philanthropist Andrew Carnegie donated money to build thousands of libraries worldwide between 1883 and 1929. Having grown up a poor boy, Carnegie required that communities not charge for library services in order to qualify for building funds. Carnegie also donated money for the 1903-04 downtown Santa Cruz main library which was demolished in 1966.

◆ **Walk to West Cliff Drive on Woodrow enjoying the ocean** views as you go. The electric streetcar which once trundled down Woodrow took tourists to the Vue de L'Eau Station (1891) at the end of the street, a depot with unsurpassed ocean views from its second story observatory.

◆ **Turn left on West Cliff and return to** START.

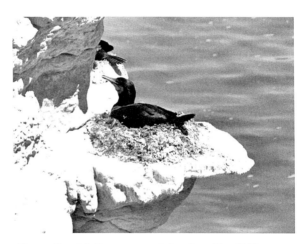

Nesting Brandt's Cormorant on ledge along West Cliff.

Reference:

Chase, John Leighton and Gregory, Daniel P., *The Sidewalk Companion to Santa Cruz Architecture*, Third edition, Edited by Judith Steen, The Museum of Art & History, 2005.

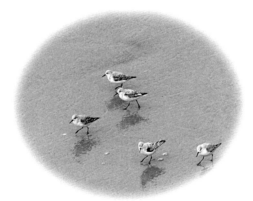

Sanderlings

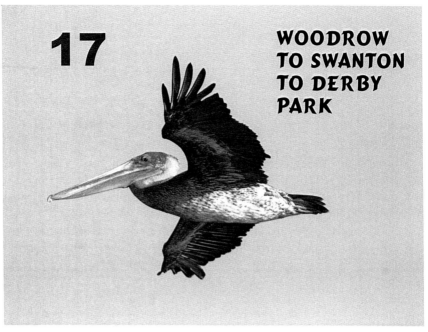

17

WOODROW TO SWANTON TO DERBY PARK

3.6 miles / 50 feet elevation gain

Brown Pelican

WALK SUMMARY

This walk explores the less-travelled part of the West Cliff path, cuts through a hidden park, and peeks in on a phantasmagoric historic landmark.

GOOD TO KNOW: Restroom at Derby Park.

START: West Cliff Drive and Woodrow Avenue.

◆ **Walk along West Cliff toward Natural Bridges State Beach.**

One beautiful breathtaking view follows another as you make your way up the coast. This section of West Cliff is less crowded than the areas closer to the Wharf. As you look seaward, scan for whale spouts and squadrons of Brown Pelicans.

As the path curves near the intersection of Sunset Avenue there is another set of stairs (Mitchell's Cove steps) down to the beach. Another opportunity

151

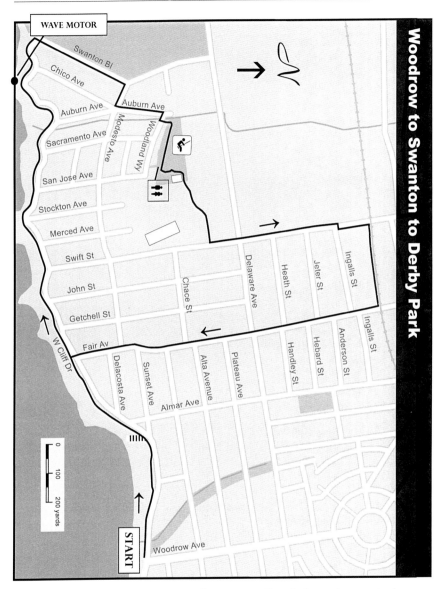

WAVE MOTOR

Swanton Bl

Chico Ave

Auburn Ave

Auburn Ave

Modesto Ave

Woodland Wy

Sacramento Ave

San Jose Ave

Stockton Ave

Merced Ave

Swift St

John St

Getchell St

W Cliff Dr

Fair Av

Chace St

Delaware Ave

Heath St

Jeter St

Ingalls St

Ingalls St

Anderson St

Hebard St

Handley St

Plateau Ave

Alta Avenue

Almar Ave

Sunset Ave

Delacosta Ave

0
100
200 yards

START

Woodrow Ave

for you to get in some extra steps if you want. Past Auburn Avenue is the sculpture "Guardian II: Steadfast" by Alan Burrus.

Peek over the railing when you are almost to Chico Avenue to see the circular shaft of the **Armstrong Brothers' wave motor** below the cliff edge opposite a modern house that juts out at the apex of the curve of the

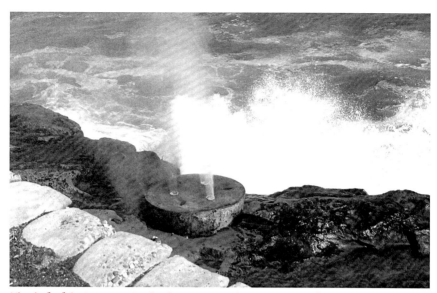

The shaft of the Armstrong Brothers' wave motor still captures a lot of energy at high tide.

road [see map]. In 1898, long before the recent enthusiasm for alternative energy, two Santa Cruz brothers used wave power to pump sea water into an elevated tank for use in keeping road dust down. During high tide and storms pedestrians can get wet when the ocean forces water through this monument to human ingenuity. In its day, the 5000-gallon water tank towered 60 feet above the road.

Black Turnstones might be seen foraging in the cliff ledges opposite Swanton Boulevard. In the spring one can see

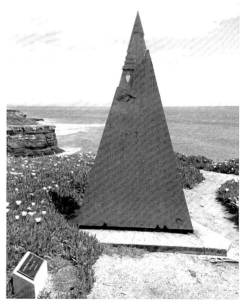

"Guardian II: Steadfast" by Alan Burrus.

Brandt's Cormorants nesting on the ledges.

The West Cliff path ends at Natural Bridges State Beach. See Walk 20.

◆ **Cross West Cliff Drive at Swanton Boulevard.** Use the sidewalk on the right side of this divided road.

◆ **Walk inland on Swanton Boulevard to Modesto Avenue.**

◆ **Turn right on Modesto Avenue.**

◆ **Turn left on Auburn Avenue.**

◆ **Turn right on Woodland Way.**

◆ **Turn immediately left at the entrance to Sargent Derby Park.** This community park named in honor of a Santa Cruz police officer who worked with children is popular with dog owners and beginning skateboard enthusiasts. Enjoy your saunter through the park which has a port-a-potty.

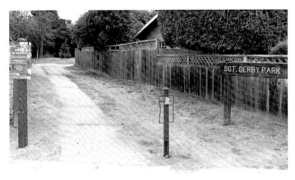

Entrance to Sargent Derby Park from Woodland Way.

◆ **Walk toward the tennis/ pickleball courts turning left past the water fountain and exit the park on a short path leading by parking lots, a mural, and Natural Bridges High School (sign on Swift) to Swift Street.** [see map].

◆ **Turn left on Swift Street.**

◆ **Cross Swift Street at Ingalls.** This crossing utilizes what traffic engineers call an RRFB (Rectangular Rapid Flash Beacon) to alert drivers. These beacons greatly increase pedestrian safety reducing pedestrian crashes 47% and increasing driver yielding by up to 80%.

154

At the Corner of Swift and Ingalls (402 Ingalls) is the Swift Street Courtyard. This area used to be industrial but has been repurposed to upscale shops and eateries. Between 1948 and 1989 these buildings housed Birds Eye Frozen Foods which processed and packaged locally-grown vegetables. The crates of vegetables were loaded on special railroad cars full of block ice and shipped all over the country.

◆ **Continue up Swift Street past the Courtyard to the Rail Trail.**

◆ **Turn right on the Rail Trail.** Eventually this multi-purpose bicycle and pedestrian trail alongside the railroad tracks will stretch the entire length of the county. It is being built in sections over the course of many years.

A NOTE ABOUT THE RAIL TRAIL

As we go to press the Cities of Santa Cruz, Capitola, Watsonville and the County of Santa Cruz are working on the Rail Trail, a pedestrian and bicycle path that will eventually stretch 32 miles for the entire length of the county on the rail corridor. This trail will be built over a number of years in multiple segments. Some segments such as the bridge over the San Lorenzo River and the section from Swift Street to Bay Street are already in place.

Future editions of this book will include more walks on sections of this important active transportation corridor.

◆ **Turn right on Fair**

At 515 Fair is Santa Cruz's answer to the Watts Towers in Los Angeles. This brick and abalone shell fantasia was constructed around 1946 by Kenneth Kitchen who was inspired by architecture of India. The complex consisted of a single-story main building and a grand entrance arch with free-standing obelisks in the yard. The thin towers are built of bricks and posed a safety challenge to anyone wanting to live on the property. The builder, Kitchen and his brother left Santa Cruz in the 1950s and sold the property.

The new owner also left town, and the property was subjected to vandalism

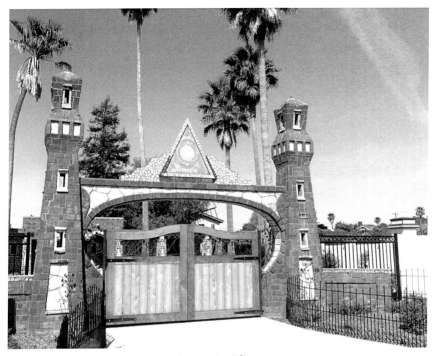

The restored main entrance to the Kitchen Brothers' fantastic creation.

and bad behavior. Despite almost being torn down, the structures were saved through the efforts of a local architect and designated a historic property.

The property was vacant for many years and was finally purchased in 2016 by a couple who have restored this historic compound as they built a modern house on the property.

◆   **Continue walking on Fair towards the coast.**

◆   **Turn left on West Cliff Drive and return to** START.

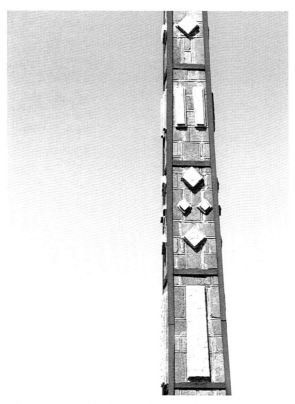

Close up of one of the free-standing obelisks decorated with abalone shells. The current owners found a stonemason to stabilize them with a cleverly-constructed exoskeleton.

References:

Chase, John Leighton and Gregory, Daniel P., *The Sidewalk Companion to Santa Cruz Architecture*, Third edition, Edited by Judith Steen, The Museum of Art & History, 2005.

Griggs, Gary and Ross, Deepika Shrestha, *Santa Cruz Coast*, Arcadia Publishing, 2006.

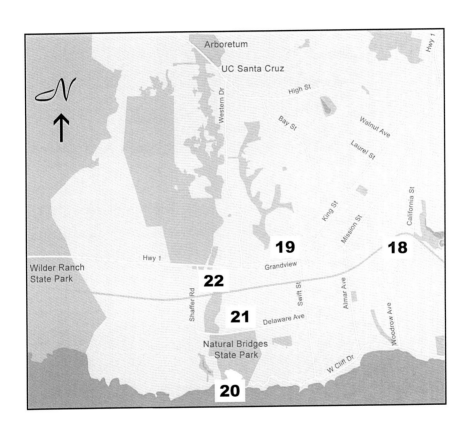

WESTSIDE

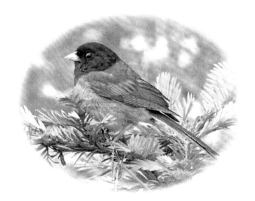

Dark-eyed Junco

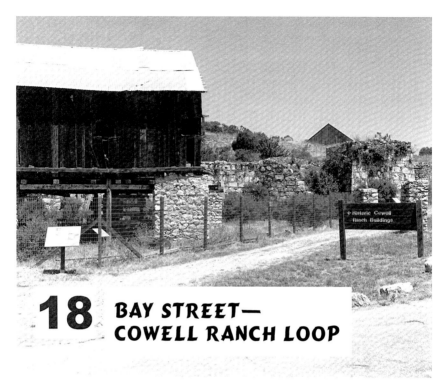

18 BAY STREET— COWELL RANCH LOOP

4.9 miles / 380 feet elevation gain

WALK SUMMARY

A hidden greenway and pedestrian shortcuts eventually lead to remnants of the historic Cowell Ranch. This walk easily combines with the Neary Lagoon walk for those wanting more mileage.

GOOD TO KNOW: Restroom near start of walk at Neary Lagoon entrance at Bay Street and California Street.

START: Intersection of Bay Street and California Street.

◆ **Walk towards Mission Street (northwest) on Bay Street.** Be sure you are on the west side of Bay Street [see map]. Your path will cross the Rail Trail and eventually go by Bay View Elementary School.

As you walk up Bay Street, you will pass two former houses of worship which are now private homes: 920 Bay, Temple Beth El (1954-1989), and

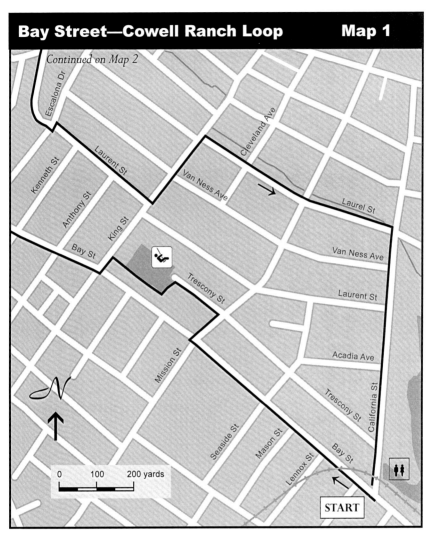

Continued on Map 2

Bay Street—Cowell Ranch Loop   Map 1

Escalona Dr

Kenneth St

Laurent St

Anthony St

King St

Bay St

Cleveland Ave

Van Ness Ave

Laurel St

Van Ness Ave

Trescony St

Laurent St

Mission St

Acadia Ave

Trescony St

California St

Seaside St

Mason St

Lennox St

Bay St

0   100   200 yards

START

1101 Bay, Foursquare Gospel Church (1946-1988). These aren't the only houses of worship that have been converted to homes or businesses in Santa Cruz. They are good examples of repurposing buildings. Other examples of adaptive reuse in Santa Cruz include the Colligan Theater in the Tannery Arts Center [see Walk 2] formerly part of a leather tannery, the Londen Nelson Community Center in a former school, and the Cruzio building downtown in the former Santa Cruz Sentinel Building. [See Walk 6].

At the intersection of Bay Street and Mission Street on the sound wall shielding the school from the traffic noise are two murals: One a 2005 fanciful depiction of a "Day in the Bay" painted by 4th graders (facing Bay Street) and the other, facing Mission Street, an ocean scene created in 2019.

◆ **Cross Mission Street.**

◆ **Turn right and cross Bay Street and walk one block east on Mission Street.** You will walk by two more repurposed buildings on your way. The burger restaurant was once, believe it or not, a bank! The Goodwill donation center built in 1936 was once McClure's Gas Station.

◆ **Turn left on Trescony.** Don't worry about the "Not a Through Street" sign on the other side of Trescony. That sign is not for pedestrians.

◆ **Walk to the end of Trescony into Trescony Park.** Here are community garden plots and a fenced tot's playground.

◆ **Continue straight on the path and driveway to the left of the garden to King Street.**

◆ **Turn left on King Street and walk to Bay Street.**

◆ **Cross Bay Street at the traffic signal.**

◆ **Turn right and cross King Street.**

◆ **Walk on Bay Street north to Escalona Drive.** The two tall evergreen trees on your left between King and Kenneth Streets are Deodar Cedars. These trees, native to the Himalayas, produce cones that sit upright like candles on mature trees over 40 years old. They are a popular tree in

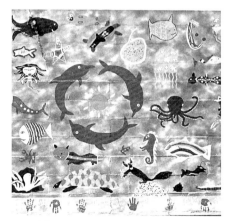

Detail from "Day in the Bay" painted by 4th Graders and artist James Carl Aschbacher in 2005.

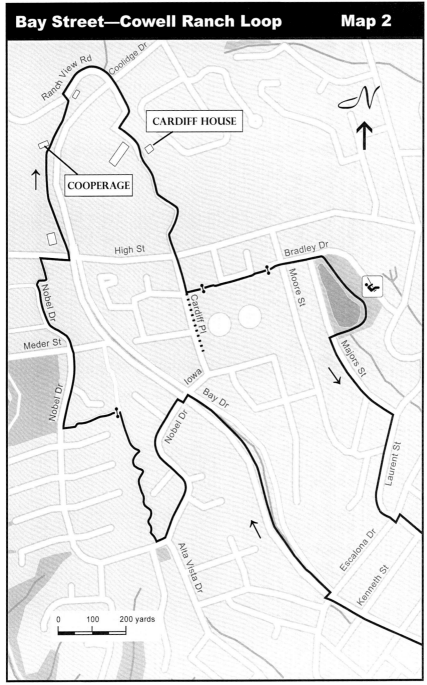

CARDIFF HOUSE

COOPERAGE

Ranch View Rd

Coolidge Dr

High St

Bradley Dr

Moore St

Nobel Dr

Cardiff Pl

Meder St

Nobel Dr

Iowa

Bay Dr

Nobel Dr

Majors St

Laurent St

Alta Vista Dr

Escalona Dr

Kenneth St

0   100   200 yards

Continued on Map 1

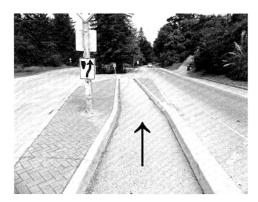

Entrance to the Bay Street Median Path at the corner of Bay Street and Escalona Drive.

California. Look for them on other walks.

After you cross Kenneth, you will be walking alongside a little creek on your left. Most of this creek has been undergrounded, but we'll see a delightful segment up ahead.

◆   **After crossing Escalona Drive using the safety (RRFB) beacon, turn right and cross Bay Street to the center median.** DO NOT CONTINUE TO THE OTHER SIDE OF BAY STREET.

◆   **Follow the path in the center of what is now called Bay Drive to the wooded part of the center median where there is an asphalt path.** As you walk up the hill, native horsetail and Tules indicate the presence of water.

Here is a blessed riparian remnant which supports native plants and birds even between busy traffic lanes and among invasive species. There are willows, redwoods, native sycamore trees and California Bay Laurel. Butterflies and dragonflies flit about. There's even a bit of poison oak, a friendly reminder to stay on the path. Surprises leap out at every turn of the path. A clutch of Mallard

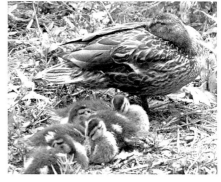

Mom and the kids in the Bay Street Median.

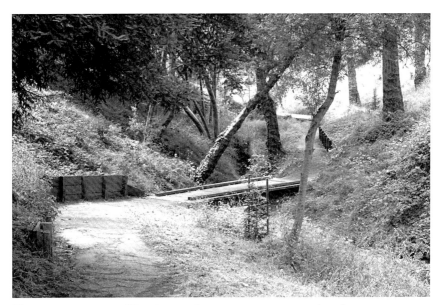

This riparian remnant still has charm and supports a surprising number of native species despite the busy Bay Drive traffic.

ducklings with their mother. Yellow monkey flower in the creekbed.

◆ **Turn left as you emerge at the intersection of Bay and Nobel.**

◆ **Cross Bay Street at the traffic signal at Nobel Drive heading west.**

◆ **Cross Nobel and turn left to walk on Nobel Drive.**

EARLY RETURN

If you are ready to return to START, turn RIGHT and cross Bay Drive to Iowa Drive. On Iowa walk to Fridley and turn right on Fridley. Walk to Moore. Turn right on Moore and walk to Laurent Street. Turn right on Laurent and walk down the hill to King Street. Turn right on King Street and walk back to Bay Street and return to START.

◆ **Turn right on a path [see map and photo] just past the intersection with Alta Vista which is on the other side of the street.** Don't be deterred by the sign. Public access is maintained on the path behind the townhouses.

◆ **Turn left when a left fork of the path passes through a chain link fence gate** [see photo].The left fork goes behind another housing complex and emerges on Nobel Drive across the street from a park.

◆ **Turn right on Nobel Drive and continue across Meder Street on the 700 block of Nobel.**

◆ **Turn right on a narrow walkway bordered by railings** [see photo on this page] next to 881 Nobel Drive. Follow the walkway around the corner to High Street.

◆ **Turn right on High Street and walk a short distance to the intersection of High and Bay Drive.**

◆ **Cross High Street at the traffic signal and continue on the dirt path entering the campus of the University of California Santa Cruz (UCSC).** The former Cowell Ranch horse barn (now a theater) will be on your left.

Before UCSC opened in 1965 this area was part of the Cowell Ranch.

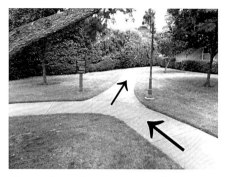

Turn right on this path just past the intersection of Nobel Drive and Alta Vista (across the street).

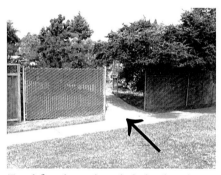

Turn left and pass through the break in the chain link fence.

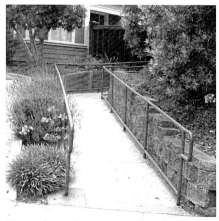

Turn right on this narrow walkway bordered by railings next to 881 Nobel Drive.

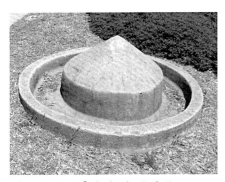

The granite pig feeder by the Cook House on the former Cowell Ranch.

Interpretative signs adjacent to the path show historic photos and depict life on the ranch.

As you walk up the hill you will pass the Cook House and the granite pig feeder which served as a garbage disposal. One of the industries on the ranch was the quarrying and processing of limestone to make lime, one of the ingredients for cement and plaster.

The long wooden building is the Cooperage where barrels were made to hold the finished lime. Behind the Cooperage are kilns in which the quarried rock was heated to almost 2000° Fahrenheit. There is much more to see at the former ranch limeworks. You can download a self-guided walking tour

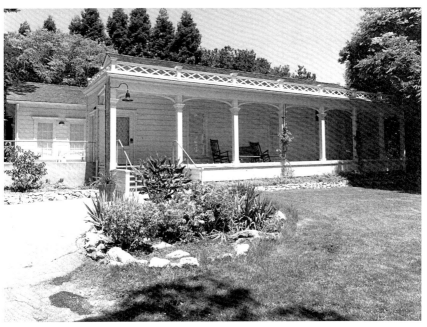

The Cardiff House was built in 1864 for the Jordan family, was shortly thereafter sold to Henry Cowell, and ultimately became part of the University of California, Santa Cruz.

brochure at limeworks.ucsc.edu.

◆ **Continue up the hill on the asphalt path.**

◆ **Turn right when you reach Ranch View Road (unsigned here) behind the signed Blacksmith Shop.**

◆ **Cross Ranch View Road, then cross the bike trail.**

◆ **Proceed to the traffic signal on Coolidge Drive.**

◆ **Cross Coolidge Drive.**

◆ **Continue on Carriage House Road following the signs to Cardiff House and the campus Police.**

◆ **Turn left at the stop sign still following signs to campus Police.** As you walk, you pass remnants of the ranch: Repurposed buildings that are now part of the campus management and part of an old fence.

◆ **Go straight when a sign directs you right for the Police.** Cardiff House was built in 1864 for the Jordan family. It is now the university Women's Center. From 1865 to 1879 it was the home of Henry and Harriet Cowell and their five children. George Cardiff who managed the ranch for the Cowells lived in the house from 1953 to 1966 with his wife Violet.

◆ **Saunter down the elegant curving driveway lined with old Cypress trees from the front of Cardiff House to High Street.** Imagine arriving in a horse-drawn carriage in 1870 for lunch with the Cowell family.

◆ **Turn left and cross High Street at the marked crosswalk. Straight ahead is Cardiff Place.**

◆ **Walk south on Cardiff to the small shopping plaza.**

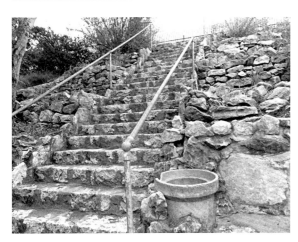

These now fenced-off steps once led to the 35-million-gallon open reservoir which held untreated water for the City of Santa Cruz.

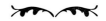

OPTIONAL SHORT EXCURSION:

◆ **Walk a few yards south on Cardiff to see the rock walls and stairs of the 1924 Bay Street Reservoir.** (Cardiff was once Bay Street).

Adjacent to the shopping plaza on Cardiff is a fenced property where the City of Santa Cruz has two 6-million-gallon tanks of treated water. You can see the tanks from the driveway entrance a few yards down Cardiff. The site was once the location of an open reservoir of 35 million gallons of untreated water constructed in 1924. The stone steps and granite walls with decorative rock work surrounding the facility are from the original construction. After the replacement tanks had been completed in 2015, the surrounding embankments were landscaped with native plants.

◆ **Return to the shopping plaza after viewing the reservoir site.**

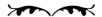

◆ **Walk into the parking lot of the shopping plaza and proceed to the gate at the back of the lot.** Public Access is maintained through this gate during daylight hours.

◆ **Follow the sidewalk on Village Circle (unsigned) to a second gate straight ahead.**

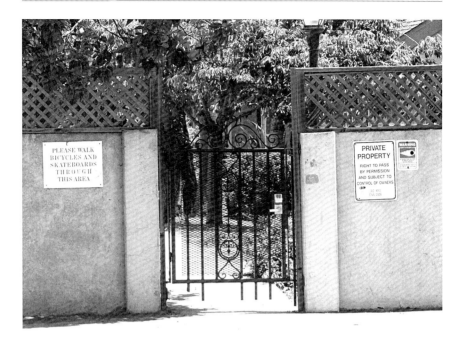

Pass through the gate at the back of the parking lot of the shopping plaza.

◆ **Pass through the second gate to Bradley Drive.**

◆ **Continue on Bradley a short distance to Moore Street.**

◆ **Cross Moore St. continuing on Bradley to Westlake Park.**

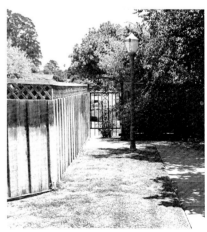

◆ **Circle the pond on the grass clockwise to Majors Street [see Map 2 for route].** Laurel Creek flows downhill from this pond to Neary Lagoon which we'll visit on Walk 10. We'll learn something about the history of this creek on this walk after we reach a bakery on Mission Street.

Pass through this second gate to Bradley Drive.

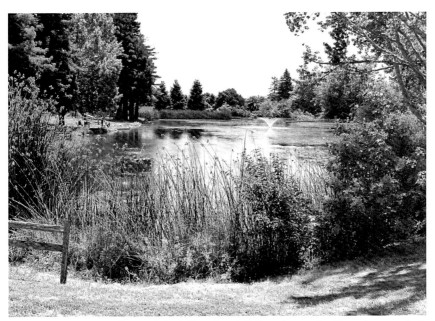

The pond at Westlake Park. Laurel Creek flows downhill from this pond to Neary Lagoon which we visit in Walk 10. Circle the pond clockwise to Majors Street.

◆ **Turn left on Majors.**

◆ **Turn right on Laurent Street and stay on the west side of the street.** As you walk on the sidewalk down the hill, enjoy views of Monterey Bay. Take care in crossing Moore Street as the uphill traffic does not stop.

◆ **Cross Escalona Drive at the bottom of the hill.**

◆ **Turn left to cross Laurent Street.**

◆ **Continue downhill on Laurent Street to King Street.**

◆ **Cross King Street.**

◆ **Turn left on King.**

◆ **Cross Laurel Street.**

◆ **Turn right on Laurel and walk to Mission Street.**

◆ **Cross Mission Street to Emily's Bakery** on the corner. Below the redwood-shaded deck of this bakery runs Laurel Creek which tumbled down the hillside from Westlake Pond. A plaque on the deck railing notes that Father Juan Crespi passed this very same creek in 1769 as he explored the area as a member of the Portola expedition.

As you leave the bakery take a look at the bakery building and the small grocery store across Mission Street. Do they resemble ranch-style gas stations of the 1950s? Guess what? They were. Some more repurposed buildings! The roll up garage doors can still be seen inside Emily's, but are not evident at the Food Bin. Back when busy Mission Street was a two-lane road, these two buildings were gas stations on the Coast Highway between Santa Cruz and San Francisco.

◆ **Walk down Laurel Street.**

◆ **Turn right on California at the traffic signal and follow California Street back to** START.

References:

Press Release, "City of Santa Cruz's Bay Street Reservoir Replacement Project marks key milestone by adding new tank to water system." October 24, 2013.

Ritter, Matt, *A California Guide to the Trees Among Us.* Hayday, 2011.

Santa Cruz Historic Building Survey, Volume III, Department of Planning and Community Development, City of Santa Cruz, p. 19, March 2013.

Tutwiler, Paul, *Santa Cruz Spirituality, Fourth edition*, November, 2012.

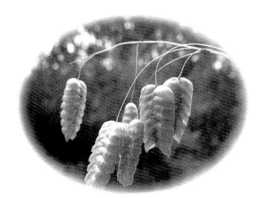

Rattlesnake Grass

19 ARROYO SECO— ARBORETUM

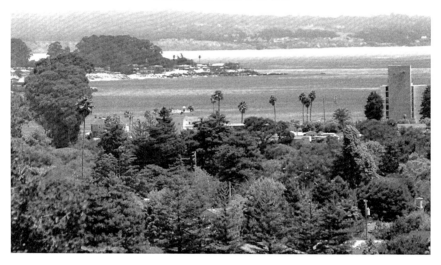

3.9 miles / 400 feet elevation gain

WALK SUMMARY

This walk begins in a residential area, proceeds up a canyon to a city park, and then to a world-class university arboretum. On the return walk there is a sweeping view of the Monterey Bay.

GOOD TO KNOW: Restrooms at University Terrace Park and Arboretum.

START: Grandview Street west of Escalona

◆ **Your start is the unimposing dirt path leading north from Grandview Street just west of its intersection with Escalona. [see photo].** The narrow path is bordered by

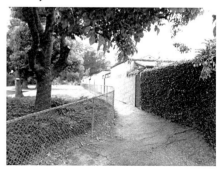

Entrance to Arroyo Seco from Grandview Street.

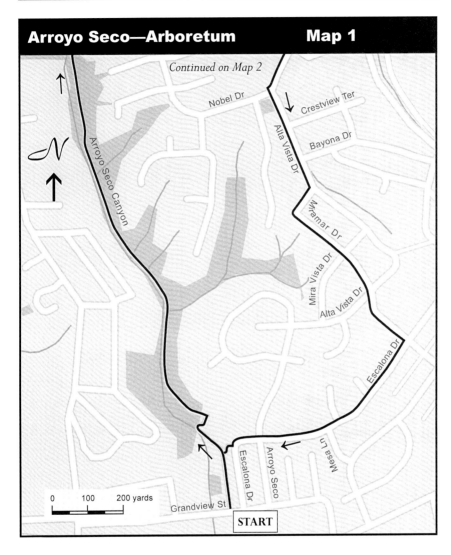

Continued on Map 2

Nobel Dr

Crestview Ter

Alta Vista Dr

Bayona Dr

Arroyo Seco Canyon

Miramar Dr

Mira Vista Dr

Alta Vista Dr

Escalona Dr

N

Mesa Ln

Arroyo Seco

Escalona Dr

0   100   200 yards

Grandview St

START

a chain link fence on the west and the stucco walls of neighboring garages and garden enclosures to the east. There is a small park / tenants' garden and private parking lot immediately to the west.

◆   **Shortly after starting you will pass a side path on your right just before a small wooden bridge over a usually dry creeklet. After a second bridge you go up a couple of steps and bear left.**

176

◆ **Continue straight on the main path bordered on both sides by private property.** On both sides there are tangles of native blackberries, English ivy and towering Eucalyptus trees. There is also poison oak—another good reason to stay on the path.

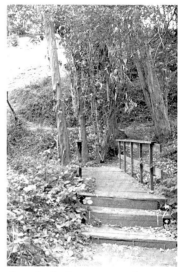

This area is popular with dog walkers and bird watchers. Along the creek willows abound. After crossing another bridge you find the path opens up. You are in Arroyo Seco Canyon. Above you on the hilltops there are houses. Around you as you proceed are delights usually found on a country lane.

Cross this bridge as you wend your way up Arroyo Seco.

Listen for birdcalls: the ping-pong melody of

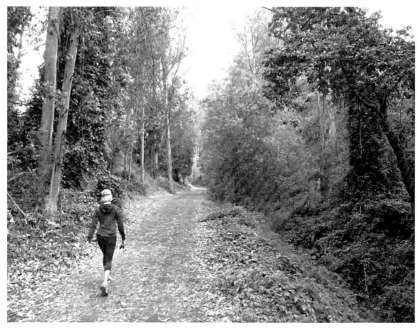

Listen for bird calls as you gently ascend the path.

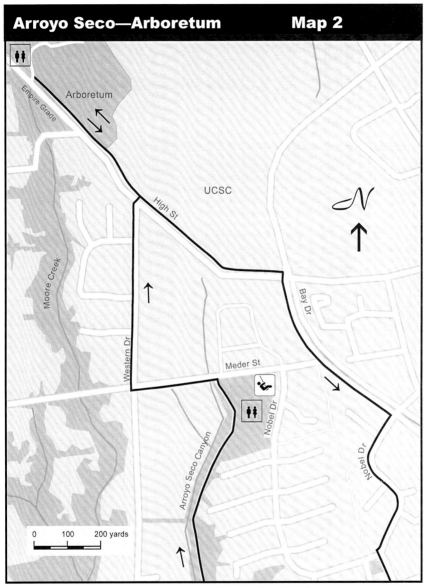

Continued on Map 1

the diminutive Wrentit, the plaintive coo of the Eurasian Collared-dove, and high in the trees the occasional shrill sounds of hawks. You might also hear the tap-tap-tap of a woodpecker.

178

Eventually the dirt path becomes an asphalt service road for one of the City of Santa Cruz's trunk sewer lines.

◆　**Keep to the main road as several side roads branch off.**

There are many interesting plants to observe including the non-native, aptly named rattlesnake grass. In the fall poison oak puts on a show with its flaming red leaves. In places the Eucalyptus trees form a high canopy above the road.

Finally you pass a dog park on your right and arrive at the University Terrace Park with its many features including picnic tables and a restroom.

◆　**Turn left on Meder Street and walk to Western Drive.**

◆　**Cross Western Drive and turn right where there is a continuous sidewalk.**

◆　**Continue on Western to High Street.**

◆　**Cross High Street with great care.**

◆　**Turn Left on High Street and continue on High to the entrance of the University of California Santa Cruz Arboretum.** Here are peaceful paths to stroll and benches to sit on amid natural beauty. The mileage listed for this walk does not include Arboretum paths.

There is a modest admission fee at this first-rate facility. An iron ranger is near the entrance as well as a restroom. The short hummingbird trail alone is worth the price of admission. On the Arboretum's 135 acres there are an aroma garden, an imaginative gift shop, a native plant section, a succulent garden, and conifers from all over the world. The garden is best known for its Australian, South African, and New Zealand collections including unusual Proteas which look like something out of a science fiction novel.

◆　**When you leave the Arboretum turn left on High Street and walk to its intersection with Bay Drive.**

◆　**Turn right on Bay Drive and cross High Street.**

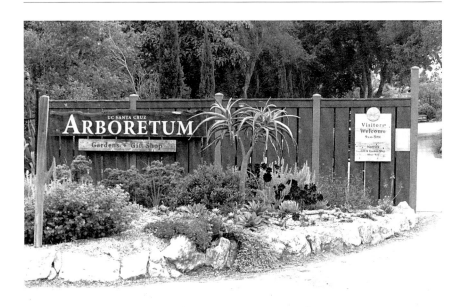

The world-class 135-acre University of California Santa Cruz Arboretum specializes in plants of Mediterranean Climates.

◆   **Continue on Bay Drive to Nobel Drive.**

◆   **Turn right on Nobel.**

◆   **Turn left to cross Nobel Drive at Alta Vista Drive.**

◆   **Walk on the west side of Alta Vista to Miramar Drive.**

◆   **Turn right on Miramar Drive. Follow Miramar Drive as it makes a 90-degree turn to the left [see Map 1] and soon plunges down a steep hill.** Miramar lives up to its name as it reveals expansive views of the Monterey Bay.

This steep hill is a favorite with local residents who walk or run up and down its slope for fitness training. Some fondly call it "Club Miramar." Go ahead, if you are a fitness junky: Take an extra lap up and down for good measure.

◆   **Turn right on Escalona Drive at the bottom of the hill.**

180

◆ Cross Arroyo Seco and continue on Escalona Drive.

◆ By the fire hydrant turn right on the hidden path. [See photo].

◆ Follow the path to where it rejoins the main Arroyo Seco path by the bridge you first crossed at the beginning of this walk.

◆ Turn left at this junction and back to START.

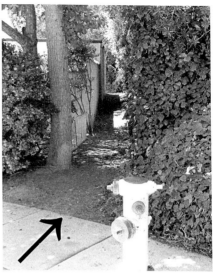

Turn right at the hidden path by the fire hydrant.

REPORT PEDESTRIAN HAZARDS

Having problems walking because bushes are overgrown or debris is on the sidewalk? You can help solve the problem.

TO REPORT A PROBLEM FOR WALKERS

- Fill out the electronic form at sccrtc.org/services/hazard-reports/

- Typical problems include overgrown bushes and lack of sidewalks.

- The Santa Cruz County Regional Transportation Commission forwards your report to the appropriate jurisdiction for remedy.

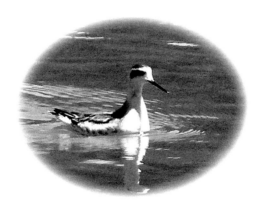

Red-necked Phalarope

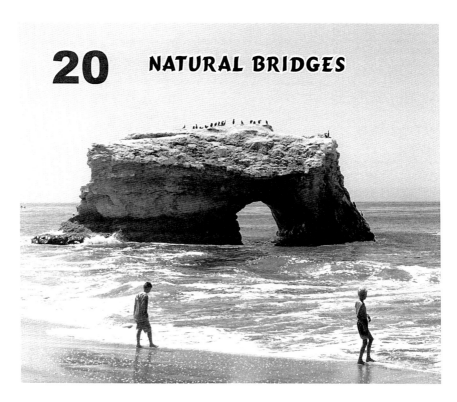

20   NATURAL BRIDGES

2.3 miles / 160 feet elevation gain

WALK SUMMARY

This walk starts at the west end of West Cliff Drive and can be easily combined with other walks for those so inclined. The 65-acre Natural Bridges State Beach is the site of an annual migration festival celebrating the birds and butterflies that depend on these natural areas during their annual migrations.

GOOD TO KNOW: Restrooms at beach, picnic area and Visitor Center at this state park. Binoculars are useful on this walk.

START: West Cliff Drive and Swanton Boulevard.

◆   **Start at the entrance to Natural Bridges State Beach at the corner of West Cliff Drive and Swanton Boulevard.**

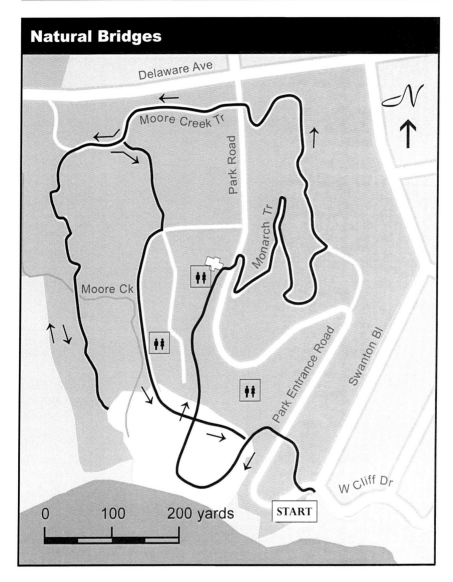

Natural Bridges

Delaware Ave

Moore Creek Tr

Park Road

Monarch Tr

Moore Ck

Park Entrance Road

Swanton Bl

W Cliff Dr

START

0   100   200 yards

◆ **Walk on the sandy path signed "BEACH ACCESS" to the right of the entrance road.** The short path winds through Yellow Bush Lupine, Coast Buckwheat and other coastal flowers bypassing the busy road and entrance station.

◆ **Cross the park road and descend to the beach.**

◆ **Proceed to the shoreline to see the natural bridge after which the park is named.** In the 1890s there were three natural bridges here. Only one remains. The waves have carved (and collapsed) numerous natural bridges along the Santa Cruz coast over the centuries.

At low tide one can walk up the coast quite a ways, however, this walk will take us to the park's Visitors Center.

◆ **Face north away from the ocean, and walk across the sand up the hill to the path by the picnic tables.**

◆ **Walk up the hill to the Visitors Center on the other side of the parking lot at the top of the rise.** Definitely worth a visit if open. Inside are exhibits on Monarch Butterflies and Moore Creek Wetlands Natural Preserve.

◆ **Outside the Visitors Center make your way to the Monarch Trail, past the fenced butterfly garden full of nectar plants you might consider planting in your own garden.** The wooden walkway leads to an observation deck below a winter roosting

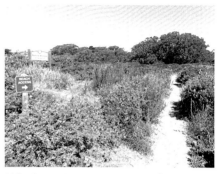

Take the sandy path to the right of the entrance road to Natural Bridges State Beach.

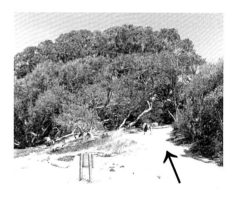

Walk up the hill from the beach past the picnic area at the top of the rise.

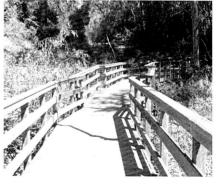

The wooden walkway to the Butterfly Grove.

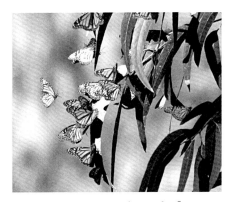

In the winter one can see thousands of resting Monarch Butterflies hanging in clusters from the towering Eucalyptus trees.

area for these delicate migratory insects.

In the winter one can often see thousands of resting Monarchs hanging in clusters from the towering Eucalyptus trees which are native to Australia. Interpretive signs tell you how to distinguish male from female Monarchs and explain the amazing story of their multi-generation migratory journey.

◆ **Return to a bench built into the railing before the**

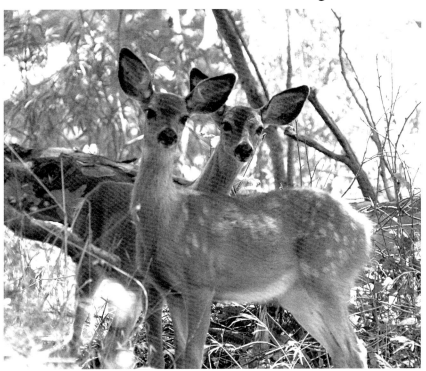

Twin fawns curiously watched us from the trail ahead.

186

ramp starts to climb and continue on the Monarch Trail which skirts a seasonal pond frequented by Great Egrets and other water-loving birds.

When the authors of this guide scouted this trail, twin fawns curiously watched us from the trail ahead. They gamboled off into the brush following their mother as we neared. WATCH YOUR STEP. Tree roots can make footing tricky here.

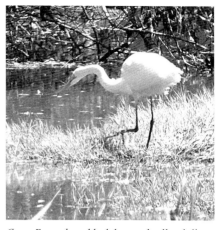

Great Egrets have black legs and yellow bills. The smaller Snowy Egret has a mostly black bill and yellow feet (Golden Slippers).

◆ **Follow the trail as it loops around an area of cypress and pine trees.** We suggest staying on the trail and watching out for poison oak. Amid the trees and wildlife it can be hard to believe that Natural Bridges Drive and busy Delaware Avenue are just beyond the fences.

The vegetation provides homes for numerous birds including Chestnut-backed Chickadees. You wander past a few very large pines and emerge on the park road near Delaware Avenue.

◆ **Walk straight across the park road and take the Moore Creek Trail (an old dirt road, unsigned here).**

◆ **Bear left at the trash receptacle and bench and head toward the ocean, descending to a boardwalk among willows and other riparian plants.**

◆ **Cross Moore Creek.** In

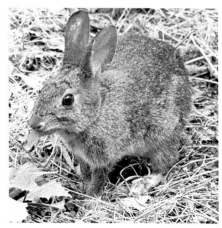

Brush rabbits are common in the woods at Natural Bridges

summer one can hear the joyful shouts of children on the beach. Soon you have glimpses of the beach and wetlands and a stunning view of the natural bridge. Dragonflies buzz overhead. Soon the trail ends at a lagoon. Be aware of poison oak on both sides of the trail.

During late summer and fall you might see Red-necked Phalaropes, a black and white bird with a dark eye patch and white stripe above the eye swimming here (the red neck displays only during breeding season). These birds in the Sandpiper family stop by to refuel on their long migration from the arctic to the ocean off Central and South America.

We are now at the spot where Moore Creek empties into the ocean. If it's not too wet, you could explore a narrow trail leading across the landward side of the pond where reddish pickleweed, a salt-tolerant plant, abounds.

During the summer at low tide one can sometimes walk to the beach and return to START.

◆   **If that is not possible, turn around and retrace your steps to the bench and trash receptacle.**

◆   **In about 200 feet after a rocky section of the trail take the right fork at a trail junction. This unsigned trail passes by some**

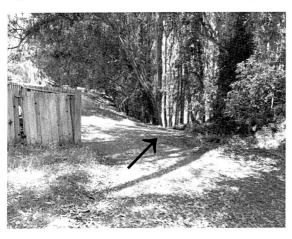

large pines and makes its way to a three-way junction by a board fence. The left fork is marked "authorized personnel only." Straight ahead leads to the picnic area. You will take the right fork.

At this three-way junction opposite the board fence take the right fork on an asphalt path and descend to the lagoon.

◆   **Take the right**

fork on an asphalt path and descend to the lagoon. Another chance to see some water birds up front and personal. The path with the railing leads uphill to the restrooms at the picnic area.

◆   **Walk past the marsh to the beach and back to the park entrance.** Pause in the parking lot at the end of West Cliff Drive for a few moments enjoying this ocean viewpoint. Here one can get close up views of Brandt's cormorants and Brown Pelicans.

You are back at the START.

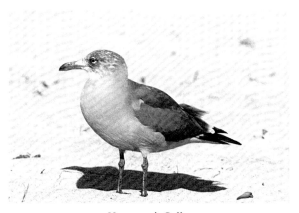

Heermann's Gull.

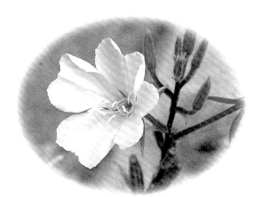

Hooker's Evening Primrose

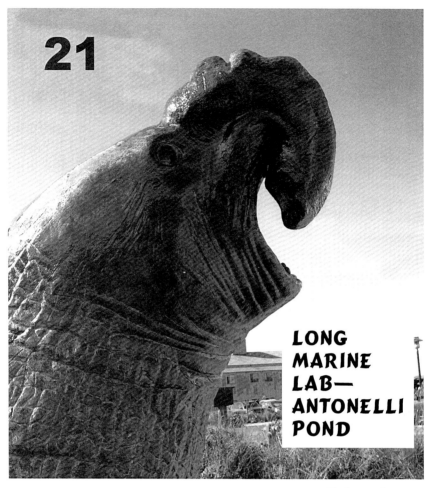

21

LONG
MARINE
LAB—
ANTONELLI
POND

Elephant seal statue

2.7 miles / 100 feet elevation gain

WALK SUMMARY

We start at the gated service entrance to Natural Bridges State Beach on Delaware Avenue, descend to the beach on a public access trail through a manufactured home residential area, and then walk along the bluff to the Seymour Marine Discovery Center. We return via the west shore of a historic mill pond. Binoculars are useful to view the abundant bird life on the way.

GOOD TO KNOW: There are restrooms at the Seymour Marine Discovery

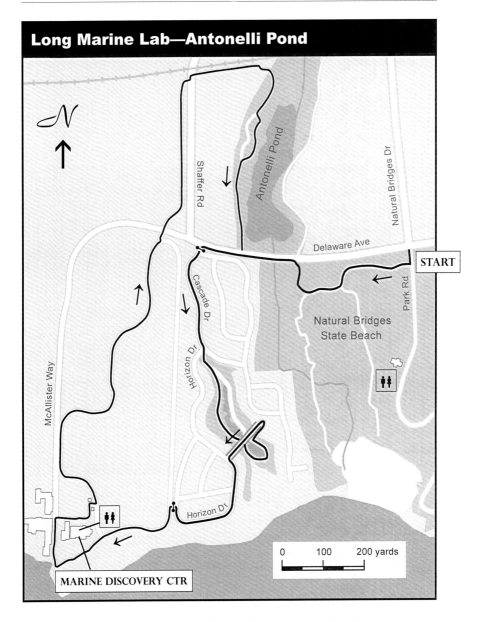

Long Marine Lab—Antonelli Pond

Antonelli Pond

Shaffer Rd

Natural Bridges Dr

Delaware Ave

START

Cascade Dr

Horizon Dr

Park Rd

Natural Bridges State Beach

McAllister Way

Horizon Dr

0   100   200 yards

MARINE DISCOVERY CTR

Center and at the Visitor Center of Natural Bridges State Beach.

START: Delaware Avenue and Natural Bridges State Beach Service Road.

◆ **Walk west on Delaware Avenue and enter the service road of Natural Bridges State Beach across the street from where Natural Bridges Drive intersects with Delaware Avenue.**

◆ **Go past the gate and immediately turn right on the trail/ dirt road paralleling Delaware Avenue.** We'll take this trail to avoid walking along sometimes busy Delaware where there is no sidewalk.

◆ **Stay on the main dirt road until you reach the trash bin and bench at a T junction.**

◆ **Turn right at the T junction and return to Delaware Avenue.**

◆ **Turn left on Delaware and walk to the gated entrance [photo below] of the DeAnza mobile home park.** When there is no sidewalk, safety experts recommend walking on the left side of the road facing traffic.

◆ **Enter the gate and continue walking straight on Cascade Drive.** The California Coastal Commission preserves public access to the California coastline as mandated by the Coastal Act of 1972. Please be respectful of the private property on both sides of the coastal access trail.

◆ **Take a right at the fork where Horizon Drive diverges.**

◆ **Immediately turn left on the signed Beach Access trail at the intersection of Cascade Drive and Horizon Drive.** [See photo next page].

◆ **Follow the trail on its**

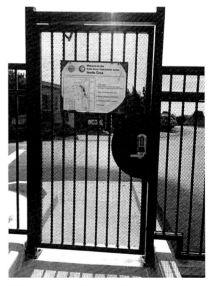

This passage to the coast through a manufactured home park was preserved for the public by the California Coastal Commission.

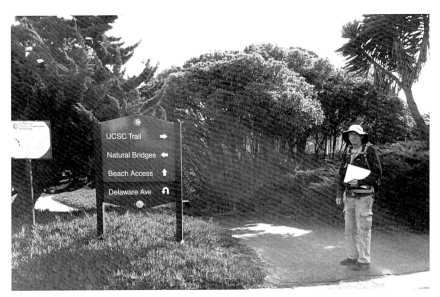

Turn left on the Beach Access trail at the intersection of Cascade Drive and Horizon Drive.

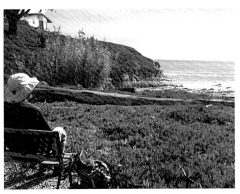

Enjoying a moment of quiet contemplation along the coast of Monterey Bay.

right hand fork down the knoll past ponds to a pocket beach. The sound of the surf can be heard as you walk in this park setting past a pond lined with tules. Soon the Monterey Bay bursts into view with a bench and ocean view encouraging quiet contemplation.

◆ **Return on the left hand fork looping around the pond.**

◆ **Go up a small rise to your right in about 50 yards before you reach the bridge spanning the creek.**

◆ **Cross the bridge to Horizon Drive.**

◆ **Turn left and follow Horizon Drive as it curves past a gazebo to a gate.**

◆ **Pass through the gate and turn left on the UCSC Trail.** This scenic bluff trail is lined with native plants which attract native birds, butterflies and insects in droves. It is a major contrast to the mostly ice plant vegetation along West Cliff Drive. Interpretive signs provide keys to understanding the expansive views all around you.

Just before you reach Long Marine Lab you pass the mast of *La Feliz*, a ship that was wrecked here in 1924 whose crew was rescued by locals.

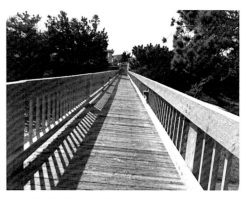

Cross the bridge over the lagoon to Horizon Drive.

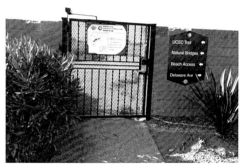

This gate connects Horizon Drive to the UCSC Trail to the Long Marine Lab and Seymour Center.

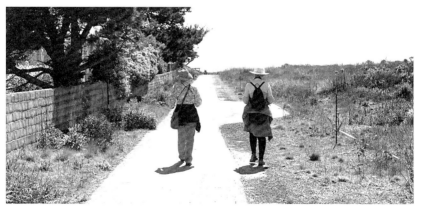

The trail to Long Marine Lab/Seymour Center is lined with native plants which attract native birds, butterflies and insects.

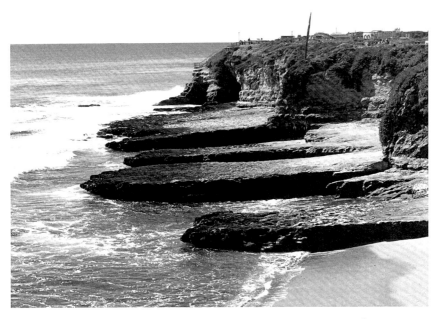

Walking up the coast to the Long Marine Lab one can still see the mast of La Feliz, *a ship that was wrecked here in 1924.*

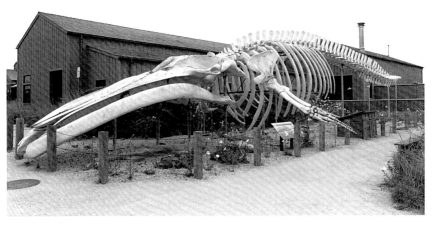

The BlueWhale is the largest creature ever to exist on earth—a fact emphasized by the juxtaposition of the skeleton and the building.

◆ **Turn right at the Gray Whale skeleton.** Gray whales do not have teeth and are baleen feeders sieving out water and trapping tiny sea creatures in their mouths. These medium-sized whales pass through Santa Cruz waters in both spring and fall swimming south to give birth in Mexican waters and returning with their calves.

◆ **Continue to the Blue Whale skeleton.** This much larger skeleton is of a Blue Whale, the largest creature ever to exist on earth—larger even than dinosaurs. These huge animals are also baleen feeders and must eat tons of tiny sea animals each day.

◆ **Circle around to the front of the building.** You are now at the Seymour Marine Discovery Center, the educational facility of the Long Marine Laboratory part of the University of California, Santa Cruz. If you have time, the Center is well worth its admission price. There are also periodic free admission days and guided walks to Younger Lagoon. Check their website: seymourcenter.ucsc.edu.

◆ **Turn left on the sidewalk at the elephant seal statue. This sidewalk leads to ramadas where school groups gather.**

◆ **Turn right at the electric car charging station.**

◆ **Continue on this path around the parking lot bearing right at the access road (McAllister Way) and eventually back towards Delaware Avenue bearing right at the Y where the path diverges from the sidewalk along McAllister Way.** Interpretive signs along the way note the resident plants and animals and the three coastal terraces which make up the area geography. Scan the coastal prairie around you for Northern Harriers and White-tailed Kites hovering over the grassland.

◆ **Cross McAllister at the pedestrian crossing and continue past the Ocean Shore Railroad sign and short trail.**

◆ **Continue straight on the path next to Shaffer Road.**

◆ **Turn right at the railroad tracks.**

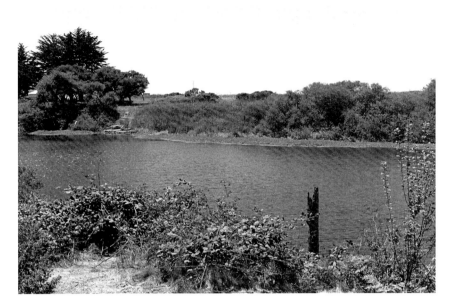

Human-created Antonelli Pond began life as a sawmill pond. Now it is managed by a land trust and is home to Great Egrets, Coots, and other birds.

◆   **Turn right** *before* **you cross the bridge over tiny Moore Creek onto a path along the west side of Antonelli Pond.** You have your choice of several paths here [see map]. Along this path and in the pond are different birds than you might have seen on the coastal prairie. Here Great Egrets, Coots, and other water birds can be spotted in the water of the pond or along its banks.

Antonelli Pond was created by damming Moore Creek in 1908 by the San Vicente Lumber Company to hold redwood logs unloaded from railroad cars at the northern end of the pond. Another railroad, the Ocean Shore Railroad, (remember the trail we crossed near Shaffer road?) ran along what is now Delaware Avenue. Over the years both before and after creation of the pond, the area was the site of a dairy farm, a mushroom growing factory, and a begonia farm. During the days of the sawmill's operation, the pond was used as a site for silent movie filming when lumber mill scenes were needed. The pond and surrounding parkland are now owned by the Land Trust of Santa Cruz County.

There are benches and picnic tables along the shore of the pond placed and maintained by the Land Trust of Santa Cruz County.

◆ **Meander along the path until you reach Delaware Avenue and back to** START**.**

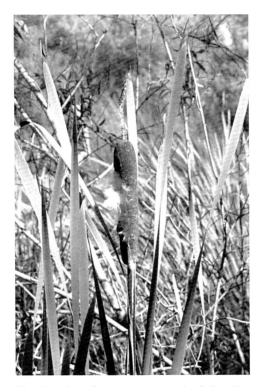

The Cattail is a distinctive native wetland plant. It was an important food source for Native Americans.

BUS ACCESS TO WALK STARTS

The METRO bus system provides a good way to get to the walks in this book without a car. Bus schedules are available at www.scmtd. com. All of the walks are near bus stops.

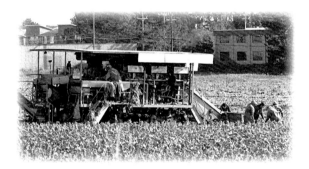

Workers havesting Brussel sprouts in the fields on the way to Wilder Ranch State Park.

22 WILDER RANCH

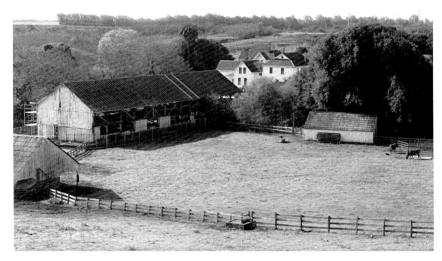

3.2 miles / 60 feet elevation gain

WALK SUMMARY

A semi-loop walk on a multi-use trail past agricultural fields to a State Park rich in history and natural resources.

GOOD TO KNOW: Several restrooms at Wilder Ranch.

START: Natural Bridges Drive and Mission Street Extension.

◆ **From the corner of Natural Bridges Drive and Mission Street Extension walk west (away from town) on Mission Street Extension.**

◆ **Staying on the left side of the street walk past a hotel on the other side of the street and down a short slope first on the sidewalk and then on a shared bicycle-pedestrian trail.** The road becomes one way for cars but as pedestrians, we can go both ways. The dip marks a riparian area, one of the forks of Moore Creek, tangled with willows and other vegetation. It is a great place to spot birds including Downy

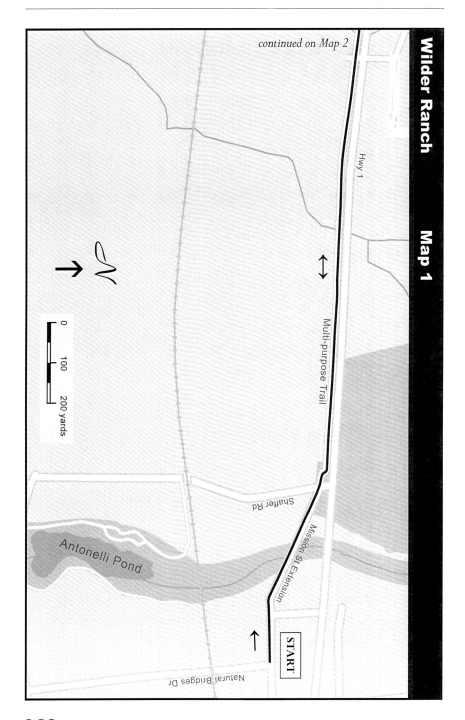

continued on Map 2

Wilder Ranch Map 1

Hwy 1

Multi-purpose Trail

0 100 200 yards

Antonelli Pond

Shaffer Rd

Mission St Extension

Natural Bridges Dr

START

Woodpeckers. The creek flows to Antonelli Pond. See Walk 21.

◆ **Cross Shaffer Road after you top the rise from the riparian corridor.**

◆ **Continue straight to the marked multi-purpose trail.** We are now on the outskirts of the city and will soon be outside city limits.

◆ **Follow this pathway to Wilder Ranch.** Our path borders agricultural fields primarily devoted to growing Brussel sprouts. These ping-pong-ball sized members of the cabbage family like cool weather and are ideally suited for this coastal site. Roughly 90% of the Brussel Sprouts eaten in the U.S. are grown on the Central Coast of California.

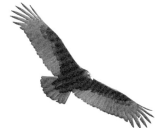

Overhead Red-tailed Hawks and Turkey Vultures may circle. Smaller birds hop and forage in the grasses and shrubs along the route. Cows may often be seen grazing on the hillsides across the highway on your right.

Turkey Vulture.

There are expansive views toward the ocean across the fields including

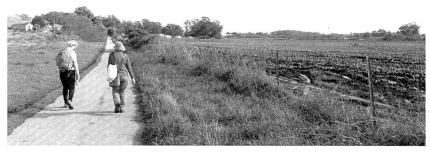

Wind your way through farm fields with ocean views beyond. Roughly 90% of the Brussel sprouts eaten in the U.S. are grown on the Central Coast of California.

distant buildings of Long Marine Lab. [See Walk 21].

You will cross several driveways leading to houses or horse stables on the ocean side. The hills on your right are part of the coastal terraces described in Walk 21.

◆ **Continue** STRAIGHT **as you pass a left turn with a gate and a Wilder Ranch State Park sign.** We will be returning on this road.

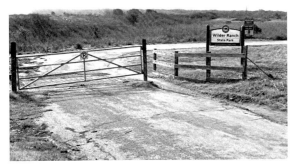

As you top a rise, you can see ranch buildings on your left below.

DO NOT ENTER HERE. We will be coming back on this road.

◆ **Turn left when the path comes to an end at a T intersection.**

To your right is a tunnel under Highway 1. Beyond the tunnel are upland trails and old farm roads popular with mountain bikers. To the left are picnic tables, ranch buildings, and the Visitor Center. [See map.]

During its long history, the ranch land was variously occupied by Ohlone

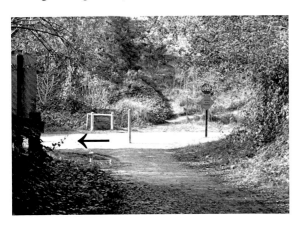

Turn left at this T intersection to approach the historic dairy farm buildings.

Indians, Spanish explorers, and farmers. Most of the existing buildings are from the 1800s when Wilder Ranch was a dairy farm. Historic exhibits include a Pelton water wheel which powered machinery and eventually brought electricity to the ranch. There are also living history demonstrations and an abundance of farm animals.

In the 1970s this land was almost developed into thousands of houses. Thank local environmental heros who worked to preserve this property and succeeded in having it designated as a state park.

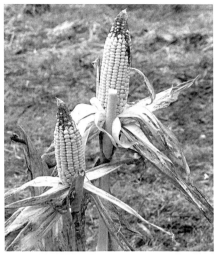

Corn cobs in the ranch garden have been shucked to provide food for wildlife.

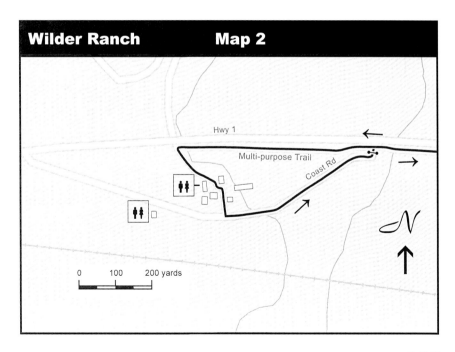

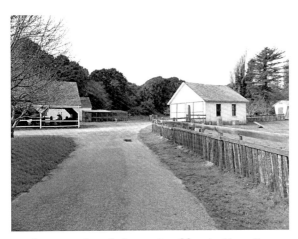

♦ **Wind your way through the complex of farm buildings and houses past the Visitor Center.**

♦ **Turn left when the road ends at a T intersection.** You are now on the old Coast Road which was the main route to Wilder Ranch

Wind your way through the complex of farm buildings. Turn left by the display of old farm machinery.

before Highway 1 was built. You can still see the center white line highway markings.

♦ Follow the road uphill back to the bike-pedestrian trail. On your left as you climb up from the hollow where the ranch buildings are located, you can see rock outcroppings along the road of Santa Cruz Mudstone, the formation which comprises the marine terraces and the natural bridges north of Santa Cruz.

♦ **Go through the gate and rejoin the bike-pedestrian trail.**

♦ **Walk back to** START taking note of the different perspective of walking in the other direction.

This walk barely scratches the surface of the over 30 miles of trails and beaches at popular Wilder Ranch State Park. Serious walkers might want to explore the many hiking trails of this state park another time. A strong hiker can walk to the ranch, hike to the top of the Chinquapin Trail and return via the upper UCSC campus.

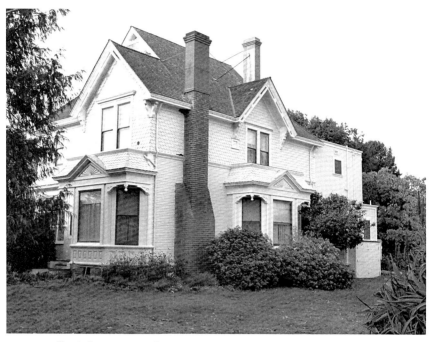

Tours are offered of the Victorian farmhouse.

Reference:

Fuller, M., Brown, S., Wills, C. and Short, W., editors, *Geological Gems of California State Parks, Special Report 230 – 2015* Geological Gems of California, California Geological Survey under Interagency Agreement C01718011 with California State Parks.

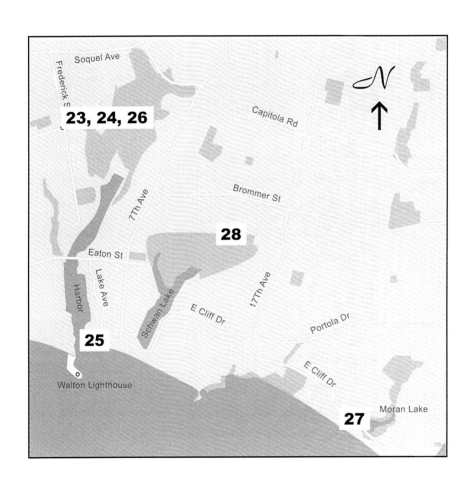

EASTSIDE

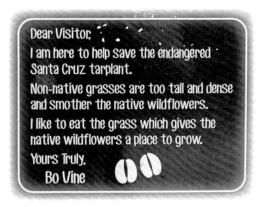

Sign on cattle enclosure at Arana Gulch

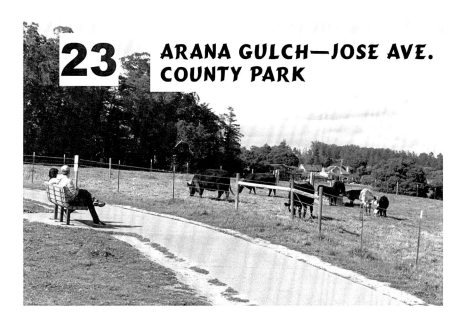

23   ARANA GULCH—JOSE AVE. COUNTY PARK

3.3 miles / 100 feet elevation gain

WALK SUMMARY

This walk starts in one of the city Greenbelt properties where cows graze in the winter and spring, crosses three bridges and uses a hidden entrance to a county park. The Arana Gulch Greenbelt contains rare Coastal Prairie habitat which hosts the endangered Santa Cruz Tarplant sometimes called the Santa Cruz Sunflower (*Holocarpha macradenia*).

GOOD TO KNOW: There is a restroom in Jose Avenue County Park.

START: Broadway and Fredrick Street

◆ **Walk east on the Arana Gulch Multi-use Trail between the church on your left and houses on your right.**

◆ **Cross the bridge over Hagemann Gulch to enter the Arana Gulch Open Space,** a Santa Cruz city park. This bridge is a *stress ribbon* design which is similar to a suspension bridge, however, the cables are embedded in the bridge deck instead of hanging from supporting towers.

211

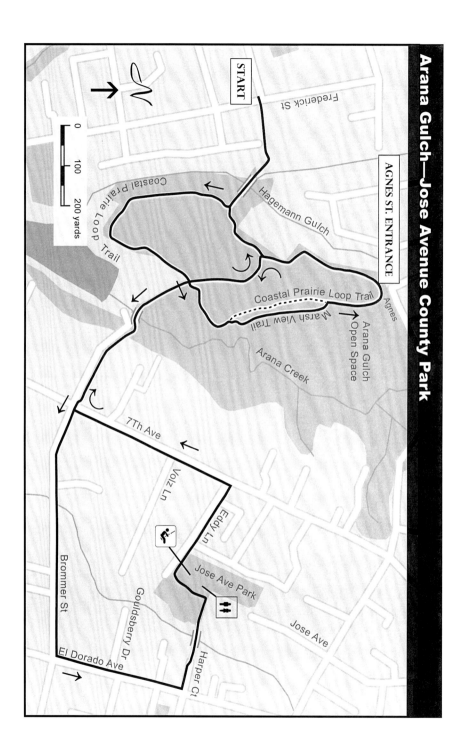

START

AGNES ST. ENTRANCE

Frederick St

Hagemann Gulch

Coastal Prairie Loop Trail

Coastal Prairie Loop Trail

Marsh View Trail

Arana Gulch
Open Space

Agnes

Arana Creek

0   100   200 yards

7Th Ave

Volz Ln

Eddy Ln

Brommer St

Gouldsberry Dr

Jose Ave Park

Jose Ave

El Dorado Ave

Harper Ct

212

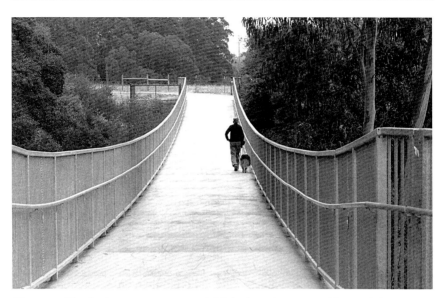

The stress ribbon bridge across Hagemann Gulch leads to the Arana Gulch Greenbelt Open Space, home of the endangered Santa Cruz Tarplant.

◆ **Immediately after crossing the bridge turn right on the dirt Coastal Prairie Loop Trail.** You are now walking on the edge of Coastal Prairie habitat, a rare meadow community that supports wildflowers and native grasses and the animals that depend on them. One of these flowers is the endangered Santa Cruz Tarplant. Once abundant in this meadow, the Santa Cruz Tarplant is in danger of becoming extinct. The City is managing this park by grazing cattle, mowing, removing non-native weeds and using other means to restore the habitat and increase the numbers of this native flower.

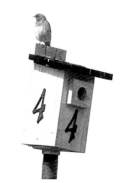

◆ **Follow the trail as it curves around the Coastal Prairie past a view overlooking the Santa Cruz Harbor.** Soon the trail turns to the north and heads downhill to the intersection with a paved trail we will travel later.

As you walk, look for raptors overhead. Red-tailed Hawks often circle above. Smaller birds such as

Western Bluebird atop a nesting box.

Cliff Swallows and Black Phoebes fly above the grassland catching insects on the wing. In the spring look for Western Bluebirds raising families in the nesting boxes erected by the Santa Cruz Bird Club.

◆   **Cross the paved trail and continue straight on the unpaved Coastal Prairie Trail which soon curves to the right towards Arana Creek. The trail signage can be confusing. Always take the right fork until you reach the Agnes Street entrance.**

◆   **Take the right fork on the unmarked Marsh View Trail to be closer to the creek.** This trail forks again and goes down some rock steps and through an oak woodland. [See map]. Don't worry if you take the upper Coastal Prairie Trail by mistake. They rejoin after the Marsh View Trail emerges from the woodland.

◆   **Rejoin the Coastal Prairie Trail shortly before it reaches the Agnes Street entrance.**

◆   **Continue your circle of the meadow by heading south on the paved trail when you get to the Agnes Street entrance.**

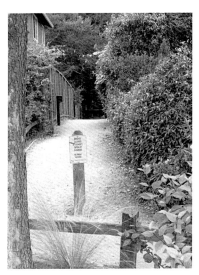

There is an outlet to Harper Court—just not for motor vehicles.

◆   **Turn left at the trail junction triangle and continue down the hill between the two fenced pastures.** You will pass an interpretive panel with an illustration of the endangered Santa Cruz Tarplant.

◆   **Continue straight at the bottom of the hill on the paved trail toward Brommer Street.**

◆   **Cross the bridge adorned with steelhead cutouts on its railing.** These amazing fish, a type of Rainbow Trout, are *anadromous.* (a-nad-ro-mous). Don't you love new words! That is, they are born in fresh

214

water, eventually migrate to the ocean, then swim back to the fresh water creek of their birth when it is time to spawn. Quite a feat.

◆ **Continue up the hill to the intersection of 7th Avenue and Brommer Street.**

◆ **Cross 7th Ave.**

This picturesque bridge crosses Leona Creek which downstream is confined to a culvert under Brommer Street.

◆ **Continue east on Brommer Street to El Dorado Avenue.** On the way we will cross Leona Creek which flows under the road in a culvert. We are in the section of Santa Cruz County known as Live Oak. Before all these houses were built, this area was home to abundant Coast Live Oak trees and many small chicken farms.

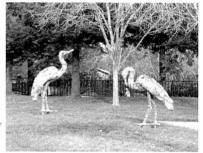

What kind of birds are these at Jose Avenue County Park?

◆ **Turn left on El Dorado Avenue.**

◆ **Turn left on Harper Court.** Although the street sign says "No Outlet," it should say, "No Outlet for Cars." Pedestrians have a passage—an entrance to a public park.

◆ **Proceed to the end of Harper Court to where a dirt path between two houses (1124 and 1125) leads to the third bridge on this walk.**

◆ **Cross the bridge to Jose Avenue County Park.** You might want to take some time to explore this park with picnic tables, play structures, giant bird sculptures, and more. It's a good choice for a picnic lunch.

◆ **Turn left on the paved path after the bridge and circle around to Eddy Lane.**

◆ **Turn right on Eddy Lane.**

◆ **Turn left on 7th Avenue.**

◆ **Turn right and cross 7th Avenue at the Brommer Street entrance to Arana Gulch.**

◆ **Walk down the hill, over the steelhead bridge, then up the hill between the two fenced pastures.** Walking up the hill gives you a chance to examine the terrain and see how different the landscape can look when walking in the opposite direction.

◆ **Turn left at the trail junction** at the top of the hill.

◆ **Follow the paved path across the stress ribbon bridge to** START.

24

WALTON LIGHTHOUSE— NATURAL HISTORY MUSEUM

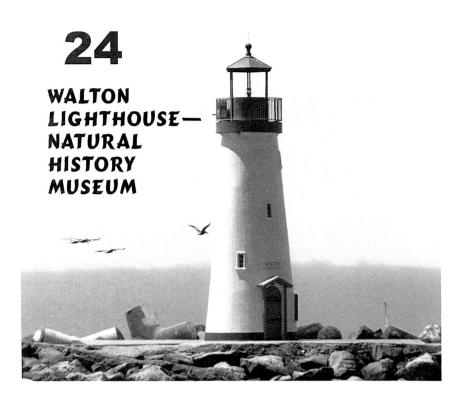

3.4 miles / 250 feet elevation gain

WALK SUMMARY

From the entrance to the Arana Gulch Greenspace we find a hidden connection to the Frederick Street Park then traverse a secret path high above the Santa Cruz Small Craft Harbor and savor views as we approach the Walton Lighthouse. We cross scenic Seabright Beach to the Santa Cruz Museum of Natural History and return to the start. On the way we go up and down local staircases.

GOOD TO KNOW: Restrooms in the Frederick Street Park and by the restaurant at the harbor.

START: Broadway and Frederick Street

◆ **Where Broadway ends at Frederick Street, walk about 100 yards toward the Arana Gulch Greenbelt on the multi-use path.**

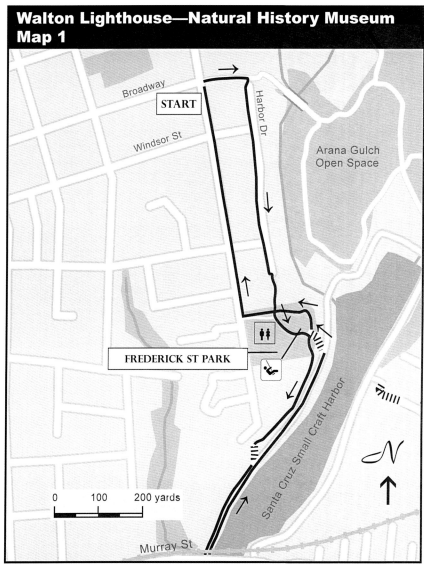

Walton Lighthouse—Natural History Museum
Map 1

Broadway

START

Windsor St

Harbor Dr

Arana Gulch
Open Space

FREDERICK ST PARK

Santa Cruz Small Craft Harbor

N

0   100   200 yards

Murray St

Continued on Map 2

Originally this path was envisioned as a full blown road linking Broadway
with Brommer Street on the other side of the Greenbelt. Thankfully, the road
was never built and instead there is a multi-use trail popular with pedestrians
and bicyclists. We explore the Arana Gulch Greenbelt in walks 22 and 25.

218

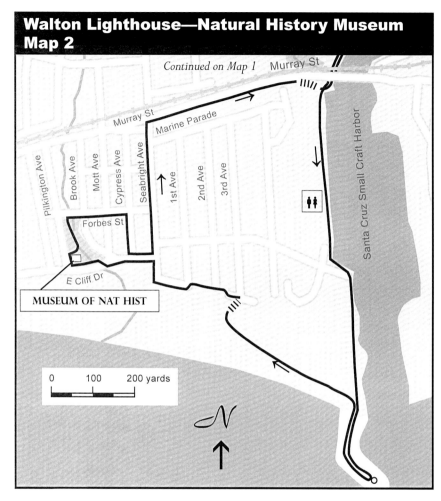

Walton Lighthouse—Natural History Museum Map 2

Continued on Map 1   Murray St

Murray St

Marine Parade

Pilkington Ave

Brook Ave

Mott Ave

Cypress Ave

Seabright Ave

1st Ave

2nd Ave

3rd Ave

Santa Cruz Small Craft Harbor

Forbes St

E Cliff Dr

MUSEUM OF NAT HIST

0   100   200 yards

N

◆ Turn right at unsigned Harbor Drive cul-de-sac across from the church property and BEFORE YOU GET TO THE BRIDGE LEADING TO THE ARANA GULCH GREENSPACE.

◆ Follow Harbor Drive to its end where there is a narrow passageway between two houses

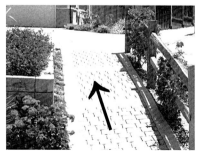

Follow this narrow passageway between two houses to the Frederick Street Park.

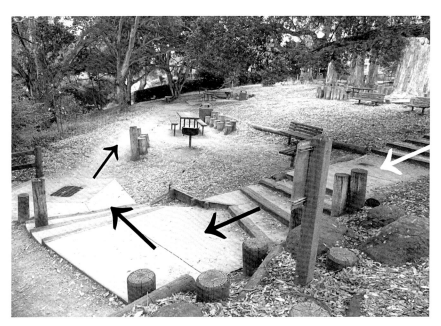

You will be turning right at the storm drain grate just below the picnic area. Be alert. This turn can be tricky to find.

to the Frederick Street Park [see photo previous page]**.** The hidden connection emerges at the park by the restrooms.

◆   **From the restrooms head diagonally on an asphalt path toward the children's play structures and tall Eucalyptus trees.**

◆   **Walk between the two playground areas.**

◆   **Descend to a picnic area and turn right at a storm drain grate** BEFORE **going down the steps bordered by railings on both sides.** [See photo above]. Be alert. This turn can be tricky to find.

◆   **Walk on a dirt path above the harbor passing more picnic tables.** The views of the boats below are wonderful as are the sounds of the seagulls overhead.

◆   **Turn left when you reach a metal railing and follow a steep concrete path and stairs down to the harbor.**

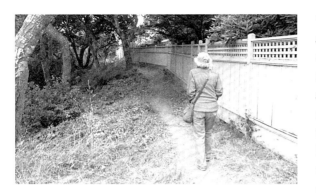

Walk along a dirt path above the harbor behind the homes.

◆   **Turn right at the bottom of the stairs and stroll along the asphalt service road bordering the docked boats.** If you doubt that everything is connected, reflect on this: The Santa Cruz Harbor sustained $26 million in damage from the 2011 earthquake and tsunami which struck Japan. This calamity was not the first time Mother Nature rattled the harbor. An interpretive sign on your way shows photos of damage to the harbor from the 1989 Loma Prieta earthquake which destroyed much of the Santa Cruz downtown.

◆   **Continue on this service road ramping first up then down under the railroad bridge and the Murray Street Bridge.** Benches and picnic tables abound for relaxing, people watching, and enjoying the view.

◆   **Continue on the sidewalk next to the docks walking toward the ocean passing the Coast Guard Station on your right.** Soon you will pass a public restroom located BEHIND the restrooms and showers for boat owners and a restaurant.

◆   **Continue past kayak racks then up a ramp to Atlantic Avenue.**

◆   **Turn left when you reach Atlantic Avenue and bear right on the dirt path leading to the lighthouse.** The more photogenic of the two Santa Cruz lighthouses, the Walton Lighthouse was dedicated in 2002 and replaced a functional but non-scenic light. The other lighthouse, the Mark Abbott Lighthouse, is located on West Cliff Drive and contains the Surfing Museum. See Walk 14.

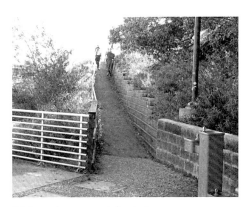

Walk up the ramp to Atlantic Avenue.

The walk out the west jetty to the lighthouse yields amazing views in all directions: West to Seabright Beach and further to the Santa Cruz Beach Boardwalk; south to Monterey across the Bay, east to Black Point; and North (behind you) to the boats coming and going. I love the jetty jacks jumbled about. The view is even more spectacular during Wednesday night sailboat races. Also notice the adjacent restored sand dunes with native plants.

◆ **After you've had time to drink it all in, return part way on the jetty.**

◆ **Turn left to the beach and leave the jetty as soon as practical.** You are now on wide, sandy Seabright State Beach, once known as Castle Beach after a castle-like building that was demolished in 1967.

Before the harbor was completed in 1964, Seabright Beach disappeared most winters under wave assault. But after the jetty was built, sand collected west of the jetty and widened the beach.

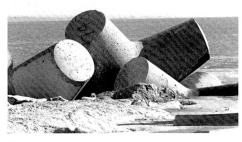

Jetty jacks.

The widened beach created new habitat for shore birds. You might see the super cute threatened Snowy Plover scurrying over the sand as you walk. Observe the warning signs and do not go into the fenced area which protects Plover habitat. Plovers can't read however, and many are outside the fence line.

◆　**Head for the stairs going up to the bluff on your right.** There are 64 steps for fitness fans.

◆　**Turn left at the top of the stairs and walk on the sidewalk along the top of the bluff.**

◆　**Turn right where the trail ends in a cul-de-sac.** This is the end of Seabright Avenue.

◆　**Turn left on East Cliff Drive.** You will be able to see the Santa Cruz Museum of Natural History at the top of the rise ahead.

◆　**Cross East Cliff at the next painted crosswalk. Walk to the museum.** Hands-on exhibits beckon inside its historic building. Outside there is a garden learning center and the famous life-sized sculpture of a gray whale near the front entrance.

The Santa Cruz Museum of Natural History, fondly called the Whale Museum by locals, is housed in a former Carnegie Library built in 1915. The museum exhibits grew from the collections of Laura Hecox, a local

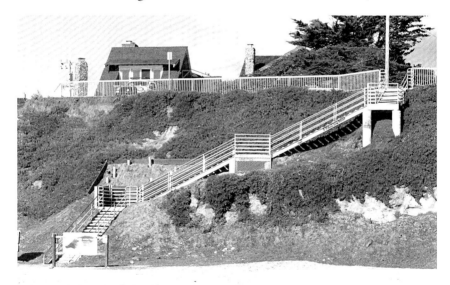

Sixty-four steps lead up from Seabright Beach to a walkway on the top of the bluff.

naturalist, who was appointed as keeper of the Santa Cruz Lighthouse on West Cliff Drive in 1883. See Walk 14.

WHAT'S A CROSSWALK?

Did you know that *every* corner is a legal crosswalk unless specifically prohibited? Only some crosswalks have painted patterns or stripes to make them more visible to drivers.

◆   **Turn right on Pilkington Avenue, and circle around the back of the museum on dirt paths to Forbes Street.**

◆   **Turn right on Forbes Street.**

◆   **Turn right on Cypress Avenue and walk back to East Cliff.** This neighborhood has a number of historic cottages. The ones at 101 Mott and 207 Seabright are especially beautiful.

◆   **Turn left on East Cliff Drive.**

◆   **Turn left on Seabright Avenue. Walk to Murray Street.**

◆   **Turn right on Murray, cross Seabright, and continue on Murray.** This short section on busy Murray Street will take us back to the harbor. On the way you will pass a retaining wall made up of rocks in wire cages. These structures are called

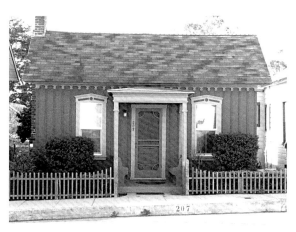

Visitors escaping Central Valley heat would flock to the beach and stay in charming cottages such as this one.

224

"gabions." Impress your friends with this great word.

◆   **Descend the steps to the harbor BEFORE you cross the vehicle bridge over the harbor.** It's a good idea to immediately get on the sidewalk because bicyclists often come speeding around the corner to your left.

◆   **Turn left and take the path up and then down under the bridge. Pass the steps we came down at the beginning of this walk.**

◆   **Turn left after passing Dock G3 and climb the stairs to Frederick Street Park.**

◆   **Turn right at the playground on a dirt path.**

◆   **Walk past the restrooms to Frederick Street.**

◆   **Turn right on Frederick Street and return to START.**

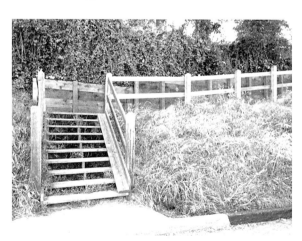

These steps lead from the Harbor Access Road to Frederick Street Park.

Reference

Griggs, Gary and Ross, Deepika Shrestha, *Santa Cruz Coast*, Arcadia Publishing, 2006.

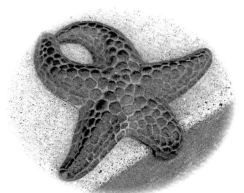

Twin Lakes Bench Detail

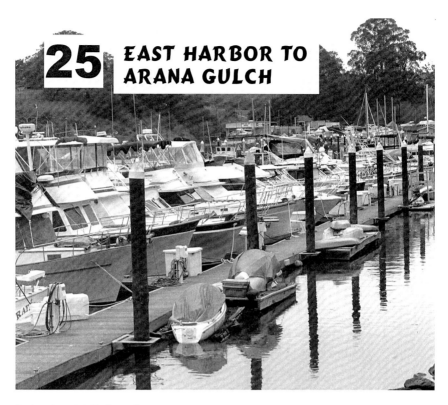

25 EAST HARBOR TO ARANA GULCH

2.6 miles / 160 feet elevation gain

WALK SUMMARY

Affter enjoying a stroll along part of the Monterey Bay Sanctuary Scenic Trail, we get close-up views of the Santa Cruz Small Craft Harbor, puff our way up a wooden staircase, and circle around through the eastern edge of the Arana Gulch Greenbelt. Our return on the harbor path is adorned with public art and informational panels on sailing ships and tides.

GOOD TO KNOW: There are multiple restrooms on this short easy walk.

START: Where 5th Avenue ends at the beach.

The July 2018 Twin Lakes Beachfront Improvement Project turned a public area that forced pedestrians to dodge automobile traffic into a showplace of public art and good design for pedestrians, bicyclists, and drivers. Twin Lakes State Beach gets its name from what were once seen as the twin lakes

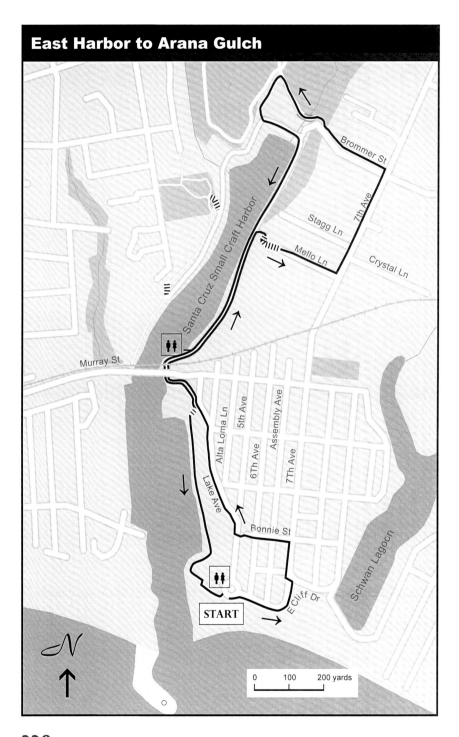

Brommer St

7th Ave

Stagg Ln

Mello Ln

Crystal Ln

Santa Cruz Small Craft Harbor

Murray St

Alta Loma Ln

5th Ave

Assembly Ave

6Th Ave

7Th Ave

Lake Ave

Bonnie St

Schwan Lagoon

E Cliff Dr

START

N

0   100   200 yards

of Schwan Lagoon and Woods Lagoon. Woods Lagoon is now the harbor. See Walk 28.

◆ **Walk east along the pathway toward 7ᵗʰ Avenue** stopping to admire the mosaic ocean scenes, benches adorned with bronze sea stars, and sculptures of a beached dory and a pelican. You are on a section of the Monterey Bay Sanctuary Scenic Trail which, when finally completed, will run for 50 miles circling the Monterey Bay.

On the ocean side your view encompasses the Walton Lighthouse at the harbor mouth, beach volleyball courts, the hills of Monterey across the bay, and the smokestacks of the powerplant at Moss Landing on a clear day. Landward are shops and restaurants urging your attendance when the walk is done.

◆ **Continue straight (north) on 7ᵗʰ as East Cliff peels off to the right along the beach.**

◆ **Cross to the left side of 7ᵗʰ at the marked pedestrian crossing.**

◆ **Turn left on Bonnie Street.**

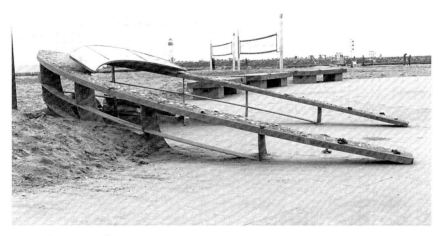

Twin Lakes Beach is flush with public art and educational displays.

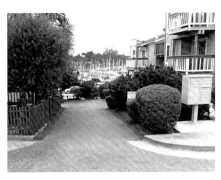

The Bonnie Street pass-through leads to 5th Avenue.

◆ Cross 6th Avenue and continue straight on a pedestrian shortcut to 5th Avenue. [See photo].

◆ Turn right and walk a short distance to the Y junction of 5th Avenue and Lake Avenue.

◆ Cross Lake at the marked crosswalk. Fifth Avenue is closed to through traffic here.

◆ Continue right (north) along the fence line to the Harbor driveway.

◆ Cross the driveway entrance and continue along Lake Avenue to the second harbor driveway.

◆ Cross at the marked crosswalk.

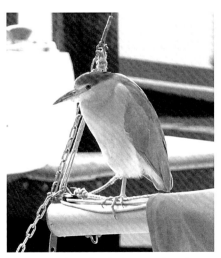

Be on the lookout for Black-crowned Night Herons.

◆ Go straight, and take the asphalt pathway sloping down under the two bridges dividing the upper harbor from the lower harbor. One of the bridges is for vehicle traffic; the second bridge is a railroad bridge.

You are now on the pathway along the east side of the upper harbor. Across the harbor about 100 yards past the bridges you can see the stairway described in Walk 24.

There is a public restroom at V Dock. Interpretive panels along

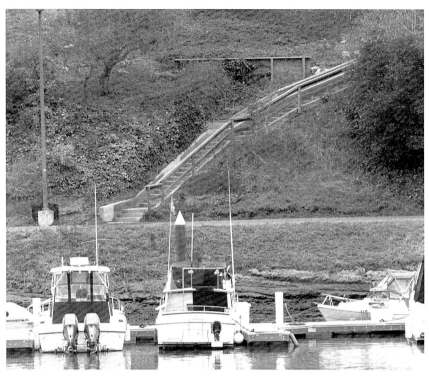

Across the Harbor we can see the steps we descend in Walk 24.

the way are full of information on sailing ships, whales and the construction of the Walton Lighthouse.

Be on the lookout for Black-crowned Night Herons. These stocky birds which look like they have no necks hang out near the fish-cleaning sinks and in the Eucalyptus trees. Often they sit on boats as they wait for tasty morsels. Immature birds are grey/brown rather than the striking slate/white combo of adults.

By Dock Ramp X2 there is a staircase leading to the top of the gulch wall.

◆   **Turn right and climb the stairs. At the top follow the walkway to Mello Lane.** [See photo next page].

◆   **Continue on Mello Lane to 7th Avenue.**

♦ **Turn left on 7th Avenue.**

♦ **Cross Brommer and turn left on the Arana Gulch Multi-use trail.**

♦ **Continue on the multi-use trail over the bridge spanning Arana Creek.** The ironwork of the bridge railing makes interesting steelhead shadows on the bridge deck when the sun is just right. Sounds of Pacific Tree Frogs may greet you as you pass this rich wetland. This is the same creek we see on Walk 26 in De Laveaga Park and near Harbor High School.

Wetlands not only provide important habitat for wildlife and fish, they also filter water and recharge groundwater among other services.

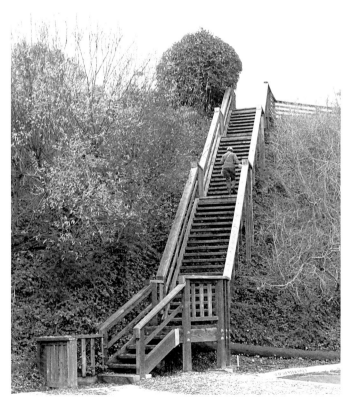

The Mello Stairs ascend from the Upper Harbor to Mello Lane.

◆   **Turn left on a dirt path at the trail junction** by the map of the Arana Gulch Greenbelt.

◆   **Turn left at the fire hydrant when your reach the paved harbor service road.**

◆   **Turn right at the road on the east side of the harbor, and walk past the RV campsites.** There are more benches and places to relax as you sit and watch the tide roll in or out. Soon you will pass the Mello Stairway.

◆   **Retrace your steps back under the road and railway bridges.**

◆   **Continue past the boatyard to Lake Avenue.**

◆   **Cross the harbor driveway and immediately descend the steps to the walkway alongside the lower harbor.** The forest of masts and nautical blue of sail covers complete the picturesque scene.

◆   **After you pass the boat launch ramp, circle to the right on the sidewalk** to the art-filled Joseph G. Townsend Maritime Plaza.

◆   **Continue to the left in front of the buildings.**

◆   **Turn right through a gap between the buildings to the beach and back to** START.

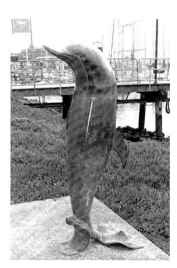

One of the many sculptures decorating the Harbor.

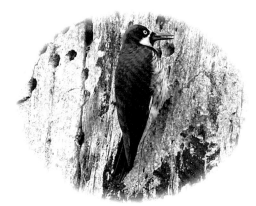

Acorn Woodpecker

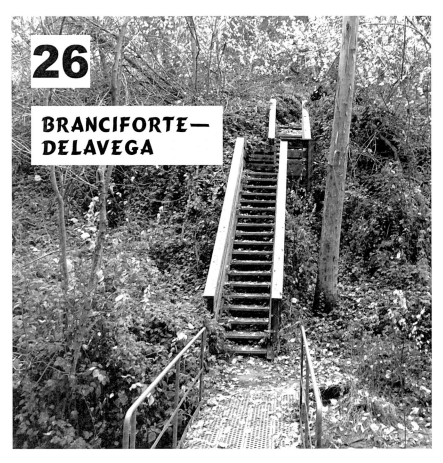

26
BRANCIFORTE—DELAVEGA

5.4 miles / 350 feet elevation gain

WALK SUMMARY

We start on the eastside of Santa Cruz, beginning with a walk through historic commercial and residential areas then traverse the edges of two city parks.

GOOD TO KNOW: There are no public restrooms along this walk. Restrooms are available at various businesses along Soquel Avenue and a short walk away from the start at the Frederick Street Park.

START: Broadway and Frederick Street.

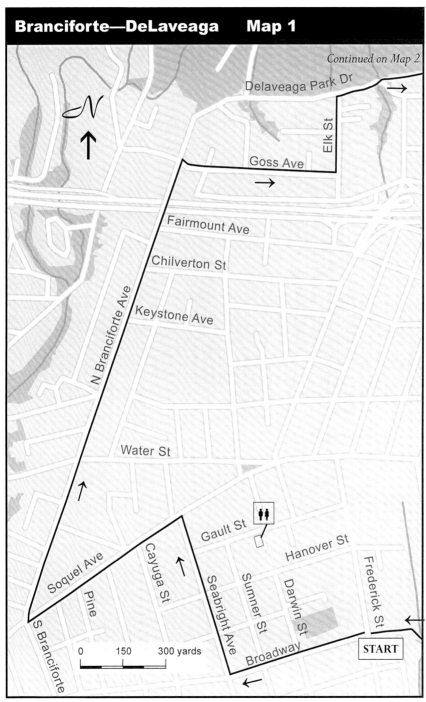

Continued on Map 2

Delaveaga Park Dr

Elk St

Goss Ave

Fairmount Ave

Chilverton St

N Branciforte Ave

Keystone Ave

Water St

Gault St

Cayuga St

Hanover St

Soquel Ave

Pine

Seabright Ave

Sumner St

Darwin St

Frederick St

S Branciforte

Broadway

START

0   150   300 yards

Continued on Map 2

◆ **Where Broadway ends at Frederick Street, walk towards town (west) on Broadway.** Notice the enhanced pedestrian crossing at Broadway and Darwin Street. The projections from the curb are called bulbouts. They shorten the crossing distance and the time a pedestrian is exposed to vehicle traffic and also make pedestrians more visible to drivers. The median island slows down speeders, protects pedestrians and can decrease crashes by up to 46%.

◆ **Continue on Broadway to Seabright Avenue passing Darwin and Sumner Streets.**

◆ **Turn right on Seabright.** The impressive Gault School opened in 1931. The Spanish Colonial Revival architecture features beautifully crafted lanterns over the doorways and iron-embellished doors artfully incorporating the letter G.

◆ **Continue walking on Seabright past Effey, Hanover and Gault Streets to its intersection with Soquel Avenue.**

Behold the Rio Theater across Soquel. Built in 1949 this theater was built to give the appearance of 3D with its curved Cycloramic screen. It had greatly deteriorated and was closed by 2000 when it was purchased for a bargain price, refurbished, and reborn as a venue for live

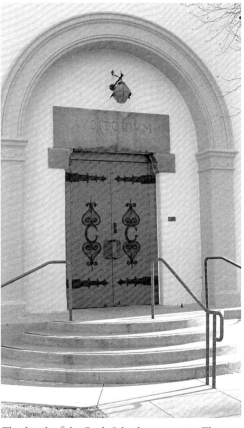

The details of the Gault School are stunning. They don't build schools like this anymore.

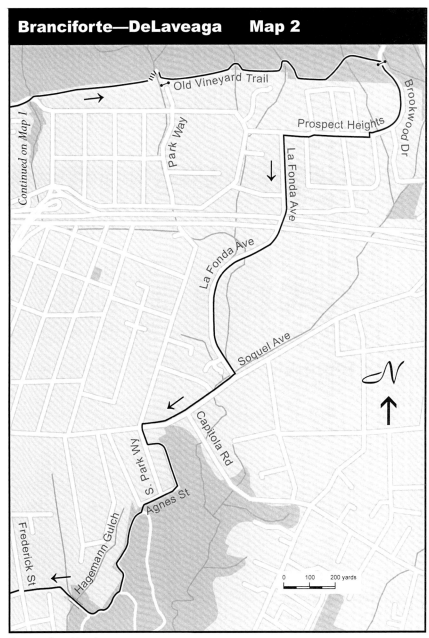

Continued on Map 1

238

performers, concerts, and film festivals.

◆ **Turn left on Soquel Avenue.** You are now in the Santa Cruz Eastside business district, a interesting mix of historic and more modern buildings.

◆ **Continue on Soquel to N. Branciforte past Cayuga, Pennsylvania, and Caledonia Streets among others.** Check out the former bank building at the corner of Cayuga and Soquel as well as Fire Department Station No. 2 across Soquel.

Art lovers, take note of the *trompe l'oeil* mural on the side of a supermarket at the corner of Soquel and S. Branciforte.

◆ **Turn right on N. Branciforte and cross Soquel Avenue.** In the 700 block you will pass a row of about eight trees with unusual papery bark to the right along the sidewalk. These are Melaleuca (meh-luh-LOO-kuh) trees which are native to Australia. During early summer they sport a profuse crown of white flowers.

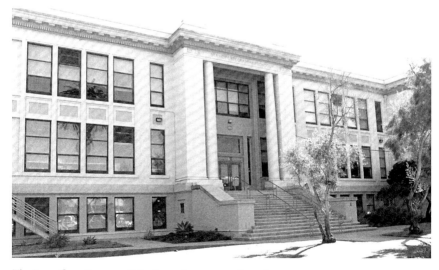

The Branciforte Grammar School now houses several small alternative schools. It is located in the heart of what was once Villa de Branciforte, a secular town on the other side of the San Lorenzo River from Mission Santa Cruz.

◆ **Continue on N. Branciforte to Water Street.** Here stands the imposing Branciforte Grammar School, now home to several small alternative schools. Designed by William Weeks, who also designed the Santa Cruz High School on Walnut Avenue, it opened in 1915. In 1917 it represented the Supreme Court in *Mothers of Men*, a silent film about women's suffrage which was believed lost but subsequently found and restored. The movie, shot mostly in Santa Cruz, features many local places and used residents as extras.

A State Historical Plaque on the grounds of the school commemorates Villa de Branciforte which used to occupy the area. Straight as an arrow North Branciforte Avenue was once a horse racetrack. Only one adobe house from the villa still stands on North Branciforte, but it has been covered with redwood siding and is not visible from the street.

◆ **Cross Water Street and continue on N. Branciforte for one and a half miles.** This section of N. Branciforte is home to numerous examples of Craftsman bungalows, a Mission Revival house, and Victorian homes. Look for the blue historic plaques.

◆ **Continue on N. Branciforte crossing over Highway 1.**

◆ **Cross Goss Avenue then turn right on Goss and continue on Goss past Gilbert Lane, Carol Avenue, and Miller Court.**

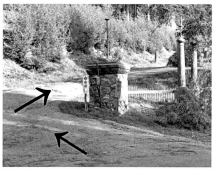

Bear left here behind the rock and concrete pillars of the old park entrance.

◆ **Turn left on Elk Street. Walk up Elk to where it ends at DeLaveaga Park Drive.**

◆ **Turn right on DeLaveaga Park Drive.** This street is one way for cars, but since we are walking, it is fine for pedestrians and affords a good view of the occasional oncoming vehicle.

◆ **Bear left as the road**

curves to the right past Sunny Lane where the street name changes to Prospect Heights. The concrete pillars you see are remnants of the old entrance to DeLaveaga Park when visitors arrived via trolley on Morrissey Boulevard and Pacheco Avenue. [See photo previous page]. This city park was formerly the country hacienda of Jose Vicente DeLaveaga who gave it to the public in 1894.

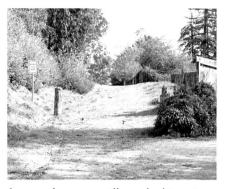

Just past the concrete pillars, take this service road popular with dog walkers. There is a house driveway on your right.

We will walk along the southern border of this large park which contains a golf course, ball fields, disc golf course, a summer theater and other recreation facilities in addition to hiking and bicycle trails.

◆   **Take the unpaved service road signed "Emergency Vehicle Access,"** a green respite enjoyed by dog walkers and others. You will pass some large Eucalyptus trees likely planted by DeLaveaga. Indeed the hillside to your left contains several non-native species brought to the site as part of the hacienda landscaping.

◆   **Soon you will descend on steps to an intermittent creek then climb a staircase to the Park Way Trail.**

◆   **Turn right at the top of the stairs.**

◆   **Turn left on the Old Vineyard Trail and walk uphill** BEFORE **you reach a gate. (Do not go through the gate.)** The trees on the hillside to your left are now mostly native oaks and pines.

Eventually you will be able to see water tanks on the hillside to your left. On your right look for a European cork oak growing next to a native Coast Live Oak each with very different bark. Keep your eyes peeled for wild turkeys on the grass and acorn woodpeckers and Mourning Doves on the ground and in the trees.

◆　**Stay on the Old Vineyard Trail until it terminates at an unsigned paved road.**

◆　**Turn right on the unsigned paved road** (Brookwood Drive).

◆　**Walk downhill to the gate.**

◆　**Continue downhill on unsigned Brookwood Drive.**

◆　**Bear right around a curve as Brookwood forks to the left.** You are now on Prospect Heights.

◆　**Continue on Prospect Heights past Burton Drive, Miramonte Drive, and Molly Way to La Fonda Avenue.**

◆　**Turn left on La Fonda and continue over the bridge crossing over Highway 1.**

◆　**Cross La Fonda at the safety beacon a little way downhill from the highway overcrossing.**

◆　**Before you reach the traffic signal at Soquel Avenue, turn right on the asphalt path along the channelized Arana Creek which parallels Soquel Avenue.**

◆　**Continue uphill on Soquel Avenue crossing Carl Avenue to the traffic signal at S. Park Way.**

◆　**Cross Soquel Avenue and walk about 200 feet on S. Park Way.**

◆　**Turn left at the paved alley 200 feet from Soquel Avenue.** This amazing alley soon takes a 90° turn to the right and becomes a lovely country lane overarched with oak trees. To the left is open space and handsome old oak trees just feet from busy traffic. Amazing! The lane curves around to the right and becomes Agnes Street. The Arana Gulch Greenbelt spreads out before you on your left. Red-tailed Hawks circle overhead.

◆　**Turn left at the Greenbelt entrance and take the paved right-hand fork.**

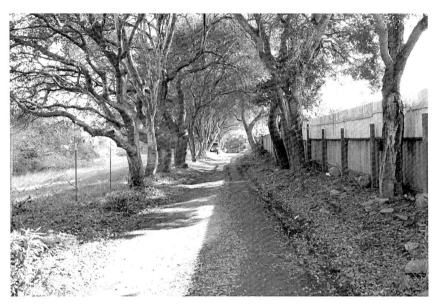

The paved alley takes a 90° turn and becomes a lovely country lane.

❖ **Continue straight at the trail junction and stay on the paved path curving right to the bridge.** This bridge over Hagemann Gulch is a stress ribbon bridge, an elegant design similar to a suspension bridge but with the suspension cables embedded in the deck.

❖ **Cross the bridge and continue on the path back to** START.

References:

Ritter, Matt, *A California Guide to the Trees Among Us.* Hayday, 2011.

Gibson, Ross Eric, "Skeleton in closet at a Santa Cruz Grammar School," San Jose Mercury News, November 14, 1995.

Koch, Margaret, *Santa Cruz County, Parade of the Past,* Western Tanager Press, Santa Cruz, CA, 1973, p.7.

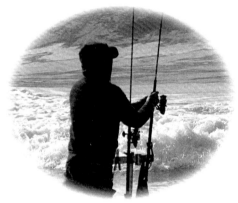

Surf fishing

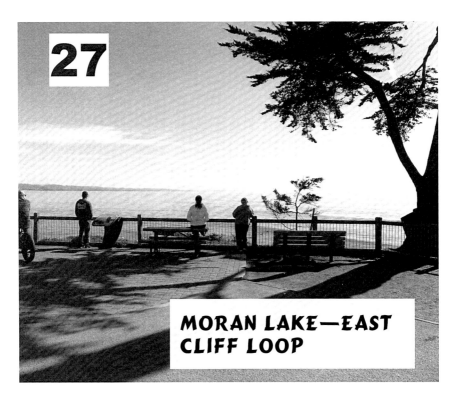

27

MORAN LAKE—EAST CLIFF LOOP

2.4 miles / 50 feet elevation gain

WALK SUMMARY

The East Cliff Drive Parkway is an iconic Santa Cruz experience full of bird life, people watching and surfing culture. Our loop begins as a leafy jaunt through a county park, proceeds through a business district with cafes and shops, and ends with a spectacular seaside stroll.

GOOD TO KNOW: There is a public restroom at the start and another at the east starting point of the promenade. The pathway through the woods at Moran Lake can be extremely muddy after a rain.

START: Moran Lake County Park on East Cliff Drive.

◆ **Facing away from the ocean walk along the dirt path on the west side of Moran Lake.** We head for a Eucalyptus grove as seagulls squawk from the roof of the restroom and surf fishers cast lines

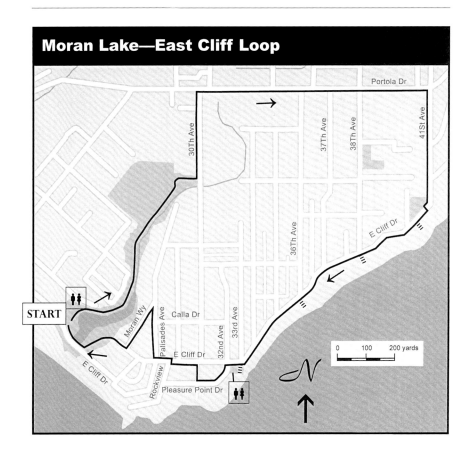

Moran Lake—East Cliff Loop

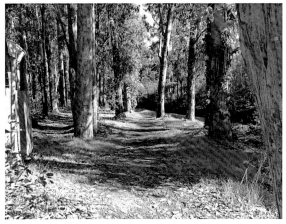

Walk through this Eucalyptus forest to 30th Avenue.

to the breakers. The trail follows intermittent Moran Creek upstream on a carpet of Eucalyptus leaves and Eucalyptus "buttons" with a scent reminicent of cough drops or herbal tea.

In winter you might see clusters of orange and black Monarch

246

Butterflies in the trees or fluttering around on a warmer day. Biologists are working hard to save these beautiful and delicate insects whose numbers are precipitously declining. To help Monarchs survive do not use pesticides on your lawn and garden and plant flowers to provide nectar. If you live 5 miles or more from the coast, you can plant native milkweeds.

◆ **As you top a short rise, the path forks. Take the right fork and continue along a fence line to a sidewalk.** You are now on 30th Avenue.

◆ **Turn left on 30th Avenue.**

◆ **Walk on 30th in this residential area to Portola Drive.**

◆ **Turn right on Portola and walk in this business district until you reach a saloon in a one-story building that looks like a log cabin** before you reach 36th Avenue. Here is a monument to Charley

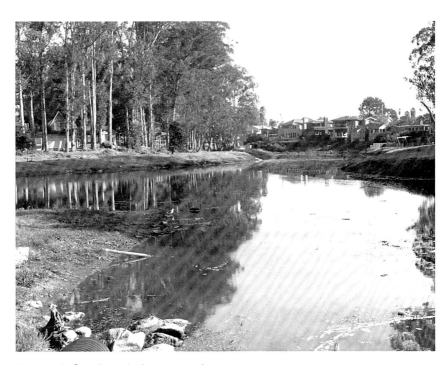

Moran Lake from the path along its east shore.

Parkhurst erected by E Clampus Vitus in 2000.

Charley's story is amazing. Born Charlotte, Charley lived her life as a man and was a skilled stagecoach driver. It was only at her death in 1879 that it was discovered that she was biologically a woman. Her grave may be seen in Watsonville's Pioneer Cemetery.

◆	**Continue on Portola to 41st Avenue.**

◆	**Turn right on 41st Avenue and walk toward the ocean.**

◆	**Continue toward the ocean passing a "NO OUTLET" sign for drivers.** As pedestrians, we have beautiful views ahead and lots of outlets.

◆	**Veer right on East Cliff Drive, one way for cars but both ways for pedestrians.** You are now at The Hook on East Cliff Drive overlooking

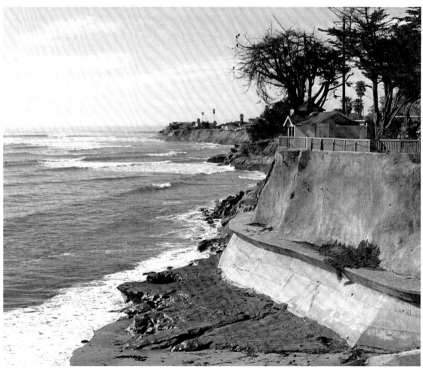

One of the many dazzling views from the East Cliff walking path.

some of the best surfing breaks in California and part of the Santa Cruz World Surfing Reserve which reaches from Natural Bridges to Opal Cliffs. If you love stairways, this walk is for you; multiple stairways descend to pocket beaches or crashing waves depending on the tide and season. There are restrooms adjacent to the parking area where East Cliff begins.

◆   **Cross East Cliff to the ocean side.** The East Cliff Promenade is a gem for people watching. There are benches, picnic tables and all manner of pageantry set before you both in the water and on the path. It's also a treasure trove of animal watching both domestic and wild.

Across from 38th Street are three bronze interpretive panels on shore birds, dolphins, and sea otters with Braille inscriptions as well as visual text. Blind viewers can touch the embossed surface and feel the contours of the animals as well as read the captions.

The East Cliff Parkway used to be a two-way road for cars without sidewalks

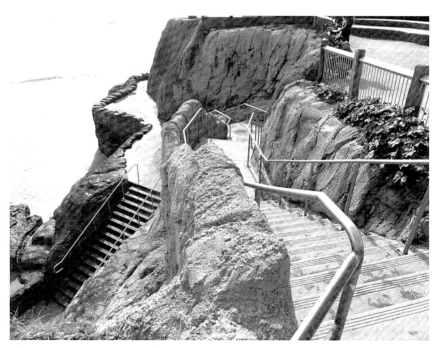

If you love stairways, this walk is for you.

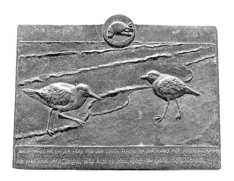

A plaque for blind and sighted readers.

or bicycle facilities. When cliff failure threatened to take out the road in the mid 1990s, the decision was made to armor the bluff, remove unsightly rip rap, and convert the two-way street into a one way road with ample room for pedestrian and bicycle access. The entire project took 18 years with construction completed in 2012.

Here one is far enough south along the shore to see the curve of the Monterey Bay.

◆ **Continue on East Cliff to Pleasure Point Park,** a small county plaza with picnic tables and a spectacular stairway that forks in two directions for some added mystery.

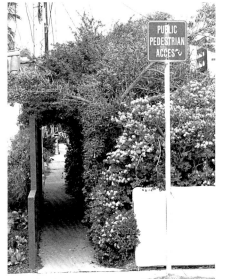

Take this hidden passage after 3001 Pleasure Point Drive.

◆ **Turn left on Pleasure Point Drive.**

◆ **Turn right on a hidden walkway just after passing 3001 Pleasure Point Drive.** You are now back on East Cliff Drive.

◆ **Turn left on East Cliff.**

◆ **Cross East Cliff at the marked crosswalk at Rockview Drive and continue on East Cliff.**

◆ **Turn right on Palisades Avenue.**

◆ **Turn left on Moran Way**

and follow the street a short distance to a T intersection where a path returns to the park.

◆ **Turn right on the pedestrian path [see photo] along the east side of Moran Lake and return to** START.

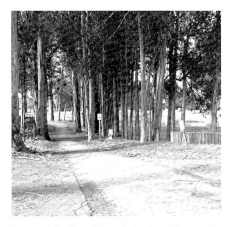

The path back to Moran Lake from Moran Way.

Reference:

New York Times, "Overlooked No More: Charley Parkhurst, Gold Rush Legend With a Hidden Identity," December 5, 2018.

REPORT PEDESTRIAN HAZARDS

Having problems walking because bushes are overgrown or debris is on the sidewalk? You can help solve the problem.

TO REPORT A PROBLEM FOR WALKERS

- Fill out the electronic form at sccrtc.org/services/hazard-reports

• Typical problems include overgrown bushes and lack of sidewalks.

• The Santa Cruz County Regional Transportation Commission forwards your report to the appropriate jurisdiction for remedy.

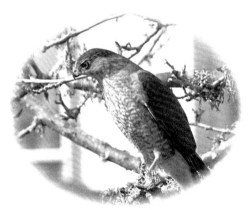

Cooper's Hawk

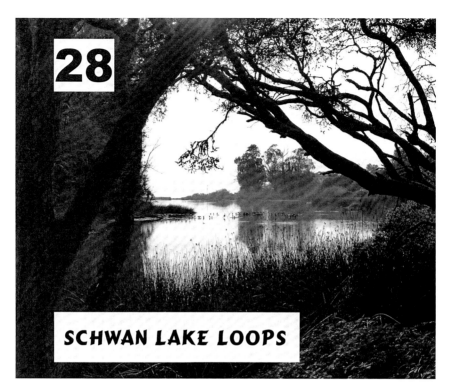

28

SCHWAN LAKE LOOPS

1.1 miles / 120 feet elevation gain

WALK SUMMARY

This easy walk begins at the Simpkins Swim Center, a part of the Santa Cruz County Parks Department. The walk itself is on adjacent Twin Lakes State Beach land although there are no beaches on this part of the State Park. Instead of beaches we saunter through oak woodland and coastal prairie neighboring Schwan Lake.

GOOD TO KNOW: After rains this walk can be quite muddy. There are restrooms at Simpkins Swim Center if it is open.

START: Simpkins Swim Center, 979 17th Avenue

An entrance sign and an interpretive sign greet you as you enter this parkland from the Simpkins Swim Center parking lot.

❖   **Immediately turn left on a dirt path and start your first loop**

253

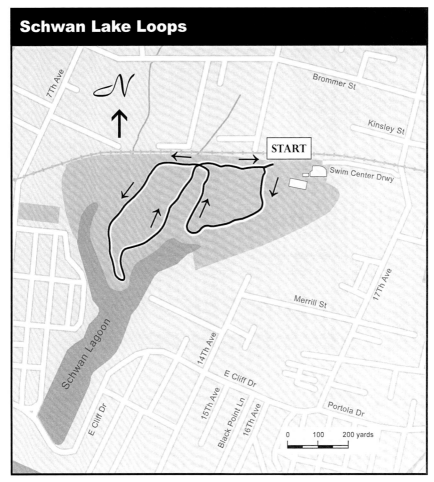

Schwan Lake Loops

START

as we walk toward Schwan Lake which is slightly downhill and out of sight as we begin. This bit of woodland and prairie in the midst of the densely-developed Live Oak neighborhood is magic. This is a good place for bird watching. Keep alert to see and hear a variety of woodland birds including Song Sparrows and Spotted Towhees. When you soon reach the lake itself you might spot Double-crested Cormorants on the water or see a Great Blue Heron fishing.

Twin Lakes State Beach gets its name from what were once seen as the twin lakes of Schwan Lagoon and Woods Lagoon. Woods Lagoon was dredged and became the Santa Cruz Small Craft Harbor. Its creation and other changes

254

turned Schwan Lagoon into a fresh water lake.

◆ **After taking time to watch birds on the lake and the play of sunlight on the water, you loop back to the main trail.**

◆ **Turn left when you reach the main trail.**

◆ **Continue straight on the right fork and drop down a small hill.** You are now on the second loop of this walk passing through scenic Coastal Prairie habitat. Soon you enter an oak woodland containing a few giant and venerable grandmother Coast Live Oak trees. Trees like these gave this area of Santa Cruz its name (Live Oak).

Soon the lake comes in view again, and you have another chance to observe water birds.

◆ **Continue your counter clockwise loop through the woods until you again meet the main trail.**

◆ **Turn right and walk back to** START.

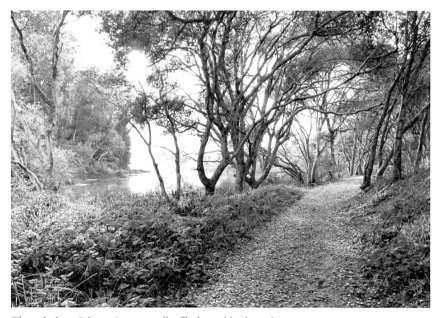

The mile-long Schwan Lagoon walk affords good bird watching.

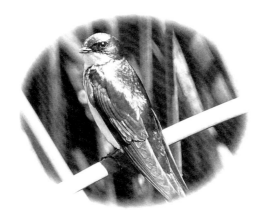

Tree Swallow

"I walk because it makes life richer. Don't let it pass you by."

—Julia Child, cookbook author

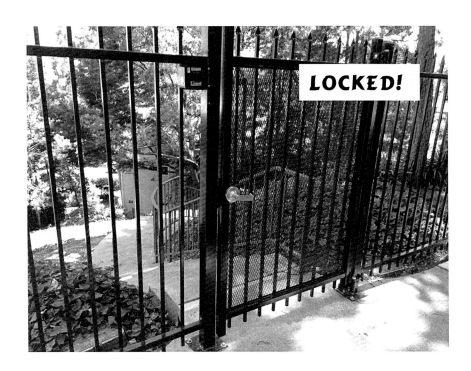

PROTECT OUR HISTORIC STAIRCASES AND PEDESTRIAN SHORTCUTS.

LOCKED!

DON'T LET THIS HAPPEN AGAIN.

The historic Cherry Street stairway in the back of the property London Nelson willed to Santa Cruz school children was fenced in 2013 and the public locked out because transients were hanging out and the property owner or city did not pick up garbage, add lighting, or maintain the area.

Cherry Street no longer exists; it is now part of Chestnut Street. The original stairs have been replaced with concrete steps, but the shortcut is still an important facility for those whose trip downtown is by foot instead of by automobile.

I ask you, would the city prohibit vehicles from using Ocean Street because of social problems? No, they would add more police presence, clean up the trash and institute policies to address and solve the problems. When there is illegal behavior, including shootings, on a street, the city does not lock out cars.

Pedestrian needs and infrastructure are often seen as less important than drivers' needs.

Let your public officials know that you appreciate and need pedestrian shortcuts. Let them know you value historic structures.

CONTACTS

City of Santa Cruz
www.cityofsantacruz.com/community/city-council
citycouncil@cityofsantacruz.com
Santa Cruz County
www.co.santa-cruz.ca.us/Government/BoardofSupervisors.aspx
boardofsupervisors@santacruzcounty.us
Watsonville
www.cityofwatsonville.org/183/City-Council
citycouncil@cityofwatsonville.org
Capitola
www.cityofcapitola.org/citycouncil
citycouncil@ci.capitola.ca.us
Scotts Valley
www.scottsvalley.org/249/City-Council
Live links to these jurisdictions are on the Lost Balloon Press website: www.lostballoonpress.com

---

Reference:

1883 Sanborn Fire Insurance Maps 1883, Cherry Street. UCSC Map collections, McHenry Library Special Collections.

BARRIERS TO WALKING

◆   **Lack of sidewalks**

It is our hope that readers will become more aware of the lack of sidewalks on many streets and that new awareness will spur them to voice their concerns to public officials. Elected politicians do respond when many people point out the need for completing missing sidewalk segments. Our job as residents is not to solve the problem or recommend specific engineering treatments, but to increase the awareness among elected officials and bolster the political will to complete the sidewalk system.

◆   **Lack of safe street crossings**

Crossing the street safely is often a problem for pedestrians. Often protected crossings (those with traffic signals, stop signs, and other devices) are too far apart to be useful. Experts recommend no more than 300 feet between protected crossings on busy streets.

Often street crossings do not have good lighting or other safety features such as median islands or head starts for pedestrians (leading pedestrian interval) that make crossing the street safer.

◆   **Lack of time**

There is never enough time. We all experience that. One can drive somewhere much faster than walking, for sure. But often it is a question of priorities. We make time for what matters most.

Walking to school with your child can provide a special time for you to talk and bond and listen to your child's feelings and concerns.

Walking for nearby errands keeps you fit and may ultimately contribute to giving you more time on this earth. Think of that! Walking provides you with the gift of the journey instead of an irritating tangle with traffic.

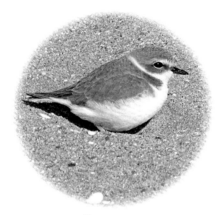

Snowy Plover

"*I walk to work because it's neighbor friendly and energizing.*"

—Florence Ladd, author

REFERENCES

Chase, John Leighton and Gregory, Daniel P., *The Sidewalk Companion to Santa Cruz Architecture*, Third edition, Edited by Judith Steen, The Museum of Art & History, 2005.

Dormanen, Susan, "The Golden Gate Villa," santacruzpl.org/history/articles/653

Fuller, M., Brown, S., Wills, C. and Short, W., editors, *Geological Gems of California State Parks, Special Report 230 – 2015* Geological Gems of California, California Geological Survey under Interagency Agreement C01718011 with California State Parks.

Gibson, Ross Eric, "Skeleton in closet at a Santa Cruz Grammar School," San Jose Mercury News, November 14, 1995.

Griggs, Gary and Ross, Deepika Shrestha, *Santa Cruz Coast*, Arcadia Publishing, 2006.

Hyman, Rick, "History of the Carmelita Cottages," history.santacruzpl.org.

Johnson, LeRoy and Jean, Julia, *Death Valley's Youngest Victim*, Second edition, 1996.

Jones, W. Dwayne, *A Field Guide to Gas Stations in Texas*, Texas Department of Transportation, Environmental Affairs Division, Historical Studies Branch, Historical Studies Report No. 2003-03, 2003.

Koch, Margaret, *Santa Cruz County, Parade of the Past,* Western Tanager Press, Santa Cruz, CA, 1973, p.7.

Manley, William Lewis, *Death Valley in '49*, The Pacific Tree and Vine Co., San Jose, CA, 1894.

Martin, Joan Gilbert and McInerney-Meagher, Colleen, *Pogonip, Jewel of Santa Cruz,* 2007.

Muth, Deborah, *Santa Cruz Through Time,* America Through Time, 2019.

Neary Lagoon Background Information, Final Neary Lagoon Management Plan, Jones and Stokes Associates, Inc. Prepared for City of Santa Cruz Public Works Dept., May 1992.

New York Times, "Overlooked No More: Charley Parkhurst, Gold Rush Legend With a

Hidden Identity," December 5, 2018.

Perry, Frank, *Lighthouse Point, Illuminating Santa Cruz*, Otter B. Books, 2002.

Pelton, Emma, et al., "Monarch Butterfly Overwintering Site Management Plan for Lighthouse Field State Beach," October 2017.

Press Release, "City of Santa Cruz's Bay Street Reservoir Replacement Project marks key milestone by adding new tank to water system." October 24, 2013.

Ritter, Matt, *A California Guide to the Trees Among Us.* Hayday, 2011.

Rogers, Paul. "Santa Cruz pays tribute to street musician." *San Jose Mercury News.* 1993-06-24. SCPL Local History."

1883 Sanborn Fire Insurance Maps 1883, Cherry Street. UCSC Map collections, McHenry Library Special Collections

Santa Cruz Historic Building Survey, Volume III, Department of Planning and Community Development, City of Santa Cruz, p. 19, March 2013.

Santa Cruz Sentinel, September 11, 1958, "Branciforte Dresses for Winter."

Santa Cruz Public Libraries, Local History Collection, "History of the County's Emeline Street Complex."

Tutwiler, Paul, *Santa Cruz Spirituality, Fourth edition*, November, 2012.

Wilkinson, Blaize and Weyers, Heather, "The Santa Cruz Super-secret Staircase Tour," (pamphlet) 2001.

INDEX

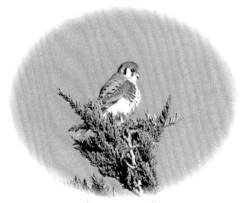

American Kestrel

"I walk to stay healthy and keep out of some rough jams."

—Robert Parker, author

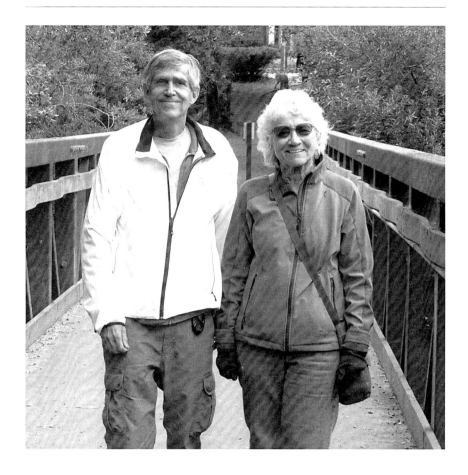

ABOUT THE AUTHORS

Debbie Bulger has lived in Santa Cruz for over 30 years. She is the author and editor of many publications and brochures including the memoir, *In the thrill of the night, and other tales from a 50s childhood.* Since retiring from a healthcare career, she has advocated for pedestrian safety.

Richard Stover has lived in Santa Cruz for almost 40 years. His background in physics and astronomy gave him the skills to utilize data from the OpenStreetMap Project to create the maps contained in this book. His photographs have been published in *TheVentana* and *The Desert Sage*. He is retired from Lick Observatory.

NOTES

1. *Combine walking with running errands.*